Understanding Health Care

Understanding Health Care

A Guide for Directors
Of Health Care Institutions

Edited by
Dan F. Kopen, M.D.
And Bernard J. Healey, Ph.D.

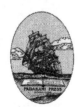

"Quality publications promoting
family, education & service"

PADAKAMI PRESS
FORTY-FORT
PENNSYLVANIA

Understanding Health Care
A Guide for Directors of Health Care Institutions

Copyright 2002

Printed in Dallas, Pennsylvania

First Edition
Published in the United States of America
10 9 8 7 6 5 4 3 2 1

Library of Congress Catalog Number
2001-135856

ISBN 0-9628914-4-4

Library of Congress Cataloging-in-Publication Data
In progress: delayed because of anthrax concerns with
United States Mail

This book may be ordered from:
King's College Book Store
570-208-5900, ext. 5847

"Quality publications promoting
family, education & service"

Contents

Preface

The health care delivery system in the United States is undergoing massive change. Restructuring will result in major reshaping of the way health care services are delivered to consumers. While there is no crystal ball available to show the exact form that health care delivery will assume, there are many available indicators suggesting the shape that the system of health care delivery may take in the future. A paradigm shift in health care will impact the following parts of the system:

Insurance

Payment methodologies for health care delivery are changing. The *social insurance* method of payment is gradually evolving toward a *normal casualty* model of insurance payment. This new insurance model will penalize high-risk health behaviors with higher premiums and reward those who remain healthy with lower insurance premiums. There will also be a meaningful shift in the allocation of resources towards promoting population health rather than an almost exclusive focus on preserving the health of individual patients.

Prevention Efforts

Better management of limited health care resources can reduce individual and population health care costs. However, this does not necessarily translate into better health for the individual or the community. Development and implementation of *preventive* health programs can help the individual and the community achieve better health standards and in the long run reduce health care costs. Health care providers will increasingly be paid on the basis of good health outcomes for the insured population, not for illness encounters with individual patients.

The costs of health care have historically been driven by the health care needs of the population, and these needs have for the most part been determined by the occurrence of disease. The new health care delivery system will recognize the fact that if individuals remain healthy, the costs associated with health care delivery will decrease.

Providers of Service

Services to health care customers are intangible and are evaluated as they arc provided. Health care services are not only evaluated increasingly by measures of outcome, but also the process of receiving this unique service is under stricter scrutiny by the consumer. The physician provider has historically controlled patient demand for services (supplier induced demand). This is changing as government agencies and insurance providers want more for less. That is to say, productivity issues are becoming paramount in the delivery of health care. It has also become necessary for providers to be concerned about the quality of health services as viewed and evaluated by the consumer of these services.

Consumers of Service

The availability of information on the Internet, by reducing the asymmetry of information between provider and purchaser, has made the consumer more knowledgeable and subsequently more demanding of quality in the health care services. The individual consumer of health care will become the key arbiter of health care quality in the 21st century. Consumers will become less patient and more adversarial in their interactions with providers of health care services.

These expected changes in health services delivery will make leadership a requirement across the spectrum of providers in the health care economy, especially administrators and the directors of health care institutions. This book is written for persons in positions of authority in health care facilities, particularly members of the boards of directors. As with any source of information, it is best examined through adherence to the *parachute principle of the mind*, i.e., the mind, like a parachute, works best when open. If you bring an open and inquiring mind to the reading of this text, you will come away with an enhanced understanding of issues crucial to your ability to serve effectively as a director of a health care institution.

Acknowledgments

The editors wish to acknowledge the contributions of the King's College faculty and staff who worked so diligently to make this book possible. In particular, the time and efforts of Fevzi Akinci, Marc Marchese, David Martin, Cheryl O'Hara, Thomas Ross, Jim Sysko, and Barry Williams are all deeply appreciated and respected. Also, grateful appreciation is offered to Brian Blight for art work and graphic assistance and to Deborah Shaw for indefatigable word processing and logistics support. A special thanks is offered to Allison Healey for her copyediting and enthusiastic support of this project in its incipient stages.

Chapter 1

Leadership Issues in Health Care Delivery for the 21st Century

By: Bernard J. Healey, Ph.D.
Associate Professor and Director of Graduate Health Care
Administration Program
King's College

What Does it Mean to be a Leader?

In almost every business in America, a more knowledgeable, quality-driven customer is emerging and demanding nothing less than excellence in products and services. Hammer and Champy (1998) argue that it has gotten to the point where customers tell suppliers what they want, when they want it and how much they are willing to pay.

For a health care facility every day must become one of continuous improvement if the business is to be successful. Competition has given consumers choices, and that suggests that the previous assumption of blind loyalty to one supplier will become obsolete. The organization that fails to cater to increasingly rigid consumer demands will cease to be in business.

Successful health care institutions demand leadership, not management. Leaders are dreamers who have the unique ability to get followers to believe in a shared vision and make it become reality. Tichy (1997) reveals a "leadership engine" found in successful companies that produces dynamic leaders at every level of the organization. In other words, individuals do not have to be at the top of an organizational chart to dream or to lead. In order to succeed, businesses require agile, innovative, creative leaders possessing the unique ability to anticipate and exploit change. The health care industry hungers for individuals who can fulfill diverse leadership roles. The difficulty seems to lie in attracting leaders who want to work their magic for a health care facility.

There are those who thought the rapid changes resulting from globalization of the economy and concurrent technological advances would not have a serious negative impact on the protected business of our nation's health care services. Those individuals were obviously very wrong. Revolutionary competitive forces produced by environmental change have entered the arena of health care. Kuratko and Welsch (2001) argue that there must be a change in traditional leadership style in order for businesses to remain competitive in

1

the new world of service delivery. This proposition also holds true for health services delivery.

Leadership may best be defined as those activities that contribute to improving performance. Leadership has also been referred to as the ability to get people to do what they are expected to do, and then have those same people be thankful for the opportunity to serve.

The effectiveness of leadership activities depends primarily on the fit between leaders, followers and situations. Leadership engenders in employees voluntary acceptance of the requests of the leader rather than forced compliance to directives. Leaders view change as an empowering and energizing force that allows for challenge of the status quo and production of value beyond one's own expectations. For these individuals, success becomes an extremely competitive win-win strategy that they employ playing every day of their lives. These individuals require little more than empowerment in order to achieve unbelievable successes.

The process of delivering health care services to Americans is changing dramatically because of environmental forces that include demands for improved quality, cost containment, productivity improvement and government regulation. These forces will not go away but will only increase in intensity over the next several years. According to Morrison (2000), administrations in many health care facilities have run out of good ideas and are increasingly susceptible to inappropriate ideas that only make the situation worse. The secret of successful companies is found in clarifying appropriate action plans to which followers can commit.

The leader must also learn to master the environment surrounding the health care institution. According to Morrison (2000), the environment consists of political and financial issues, shortages of skilled workers, physician challenges to authority, and consumer demands. These changes can no longer be successfully handled through traditionally hierarchical bureaucratic channels. Such organizational structures are too rigid to allow the flexibility needed to successfully adapt to opportunities in the rapidly changing environment.

While insurers are demanding stricter cost containment and consumers are demanding higher quality, the American health care system is in crisis. This crisis can produce opportunities if transformational leadership emerges from the administration and the Board of Directors of health care facilities. This leadership will require the building of a thick culture of cooperation among employees and the need for conflict management skills as the pace of change accelerates.

Leaders also require power to influence employers to become loyal followers. Daft (2001) found several types of power evident in organizations. These types of power include: legitimate, reward, coercive, charisma and expertise. The first three types of power, i.e., legitimate, reward and coercive, are extrinsic and granted to a manager by the organization. Extrinsic powers can be taken away by the organization. These powers do not work very well in a changing organization. The best source of power for leaders is found in their expertise (the abilities that are valued in the current environment) and in the gift of charisma (the hard to define but easily recognizable capacity to rally followers towards goal achievement).

Charisma and expertise reside in the individual and cannot be taken away by the organization. These intrinsic powers allow the leader to be creative and take risks he or she would not take if totally dependent on the organization for future employment. These powers also allow an individual to lead by genuinely empowering followers to take their own risks and grow along with the leader. When leaders and followers are empowered, creativity thrives and synergy becomes the norm.

Leadership is a narrower concept than is management, and leadership can to a significant degree be developed through training. Once leadership skills are developed, they need to be practiced or they will deteriorate rapidly. Tichy (1997) found that many companies exist in a state of wandering from crisis to crisis and never develop self-awareness of this ineffectual dilemma. He proposed that the solution to this crisis-to-crisis existence lies in the creation of a leadership engine that creates dynamic leaders at every level of the organization. Drucker (1999) believes leaders and followers in institutions have to take community responsibility beyond the walls of their own institution.

A healthy community requires that there be collaboration with other agencies and leaders' involvement in the broader pursuit of general community health. According to the Centers for Disease Control and Prevention (1995), this goal might be accomplished by combining the expertise of public health agencies and the resources of managed care. The track record to date has been less than impressive as the ability to pursue long-term objectives suffers at the hands of short-term financial expediencies.

Why Culture is Important to Health Services Institutions

The culture of a company consists of a mix of values, beliefs, and attitudes that are held in common by the majority of the members of an organization. A thick positive culture directed toward continuous improvement allows talented people to work together in the pursuit of the goal of satisfying the customer. Thick culture plays a critical role in the ability of a leader to create a shared vision. The culture of a company includes everything transactional including language, ceremonies and rituals. Among the most important components of culture are the daily encounters in the working environment and the respect for all persons that exists at this level of person-to-person interaction.

The building of a health care delivery team with a thick positive culture is one of the most important roles for the leader of the organization. A thick culture nurtures the emergence and growth of commitment among followers. This in turn allows organizational goals to be achieved. Thick cultures allow development and growth in the business through teamwork.

Organizational values are paramount in the shaping of the company culture. Daft (2001) found culture to include enduring values that have worth and add value to the organization. It is important to realize that these values can vary in different parts of the organization, but the more important institutional values must be found throughout the business. The best run companies in the world have core values that are accepted by all employees. Therefore, the leader's job includes espousing the values that are important and explaining in words and actions the importance of these core values to future success. The way employees expect to be and are treated by the administration is vital to the development of a strong positive culture where company goals and employee goals are shared. A culture of continuous improvement on a daily basis is necessary for the survival of health care facilities. The changing health care environment is producing opportunities but it is also producing new competitors. This competition will result in excellent companies surviving and less-than-excellent companies failing.

The culture of a company is formed over a long period of time and is very difficult to change by fiat. Once accepted by the majority of employees' culture not only reflects but also generates employee expectations. Culture can be differ across departments of the company as a result of leadership styles in the various departments. Because of the centrality of culture to the functioning of the organization, the first task that should be undertaken by a new leader is a culture audit.

4

A culture audit will usually reveal both the level of commitment to company goals by employees and the thickness of the current culture. The leader should then prepare an action plan to strengthen and mold the culture to suit the goals being pursued by the health care facility. As crucial as a culture audit is to the success of new leadership, culture audits are not usually performed, are most often done ineffectively when they are undertaken, and are rarely formally reported to the board.

The Boards of Directors of health care facilities need to become committed to quality at the source of delivery. There must be a demand for one hundred percent satisfaction by the consumer. This level of satisfaction will not only retain current customers, but will allow the facility to increase the customer base through word-of-mouth, which remains the most effective means of promotion in the health care marketplace. This commitment to the delivery of excellent service requires empowerment of the total employee base.

The most important assignment that the board delegates to administrators of health facilities is that of culture building. Establishing and nurturing a healthy culture is a difficult task because it takes time to develop trust among the employees. Trust is a necessary component for building a committed team. Because of the need to build trust over time, building a thick positive culture cannot occur in an organization where turnover is so high that the revolving door precludes trust building. Directors need to have an understanding of institutional turnover. The Board of Directors needs to determine company values, make them part of the mission statement, and require administrators through words and actions to constantly communicate these values to all employees. Board leadership in culture building will determine the success or failure of the health care facility as it moves into the turbulent world of constant change.

On the other hand, recent research has uncovered the fact that very strong cultures can sometimes work against the business. Kotter and Heskett (1992) provide a convincing argument that although strong corporate cultures can create excellent business production and profits, successful performance can also allow the emergence of arrogance. Some very good companies have become predominantly inwardly focused allowing rigid bureaucracies to develop, thus undermining the ability to adapt to future change. Organizations marked by thin cultures will usually suffer from poor performance. Performance problems will be reflected in future negative financial impact. It becomes the leaders' responsibility to monitor the culture, making certain that appropriate change is accepted and encouraged. The vision should be communicated on a daily basis to followers. Aspects of both cheerleading and offering of appropriate incentives may be used to motivate followers to behave like leaders when and where appropriate.

The Process of Change and the Need for Conflict Management

Change is an inevitable part of redesign efforts and most often results in chaos and resistance. Historically the health care industry has resisted change. This in large part is due to the fact that the demand for most health services has been inelastic. Inelastic demand is reflected in the stability of demand for services despite rising prices for those services. This scenario is made possible by the perceived necessity of those services. The heavily bureaucratic health industry has not only been allowed to waste scarce community resources but it has been and continues to be rewarded for costly mistakes in the allocation of health resources. Excess capacity has traditionally not been a barrier to decisions to invest in bricks and mortar projects in efforts to enhance institutional prestige. There are increasing pressures to not tolerate such wasteful mistakes in the emerging health care delivery system. The acknowledged and growing scarcity of resources and stricter consumer expectations of efficiencies in health care delivery will result in greater scrutiny of institutional spending habits. While the increasingly informed consumer will demand excellence in the receipt of health services, it will be incumbent upon boards of directors to understand both economies of scale and economies of scope before committing to expensive projects and duplicative services. Profligate spending by administrators and boards will have to be restrained through recognition that there are services that are both better provided and at lower costs outside of one's own the institution. This will not be achieved through bureaucratic governmental oversight. The failure of certificate of need (CON) programs speaks to the unworkability of politicized solutions to what are fundamentally ethical problems.

Environmental forces are also changing the way health services are delivered to the population in the United States. This trillion-dollar plus per year business is clearly at a crossroads as it moves into the new century. The change process requires a sense of urgency in responding to the turbulent world of health services delivery. This is not the time to resist change, but rather to produce a flexible organization that can appropriately respond in a timely fashion to the changes wrought by environmental factors.

Profound demographic changes are also in progress. Increased life expectancy for Americans is one of the major environmental changes. The life expectancy of Americans has dramatically increased over the last hundred years, and this is mainly due to the successes of public health

6

programs. Although this is good news in most respects, increased longevity is posing new questions and challenges for the allocation of health care resources. A large number of older Americans are coming to the health care system with chronic diseases that cannot be cured, only managed. Many of these chronic diseases have been caused by individual choice to engage in high-risk behaviors. Many behaviors that are destructive of health could have been avoided if the health system had in place a different insurance premium paradigm for health care expense coverage.

The social model of insurance, wherein there is no premium paid for choosing high-risk behaviors, is gradually being challenged by a more realistic casualty model of payment as is the norm in most other types of insurance coverage. This change will require a much different emphasis in the way health services are delivered in this country. The role of health services facilities will gradually evolve to place increasing emphasis on keeping populations healthy and preventing illness.

Change in the method of insurance payment, a more informed and demanding consumer, and the need to move beyond the walls of the institution are going to prompt major changes in the delivery of health care services. Initial stages of the change process are usually attended by resistance and confusion, but if managed properly the result can be integration and commitment. Challenges to the business-as-usual standard of health care delivery have already produced tremendous conflict among health care employees. This conflict is in large part a result of the inability of administrators and board members to recognize and adapt to the changing health care environment.

It becomes the responsibility of leadership to educate employees with respect to ongoing and upcoming change. This includes the need to effectively communicate the reasons driving change. The leader must establish a sense of urgency among employees to learn about and embrace change and to eventually anchor the results of the change in the culture of the organization. The speed of change, largely a reflection of technological advances, is forcing employees to learn whole new ways of doing their jobs. Followers need to be involved in change, properly trained for change, and given concrete incentives to embrace change.

Conflict

Bureaucratic industries usually view conflict as undesirable and attempt to suppress conflict through the application of increasingly rigid rules and exacting policies. In fact, in a bureaucracy, those causing conflict are often

7

disciplined and soon learn that conflict is not wanted and may not be tolerated in the organization. Unfortunately, those causing conflict are often the most innovative and creative employees found in the company. Since their ideas are not valued by the organization, these persons often seek employment with firms that tolerate mavericks.

Today, conflict is a given, especially in organizations dealing with restructuring. Research has shown that conflict can result in hostility and withdrawal by some employees, but in other employees the results can be increased motivation and improved performance. The new view of conflict is that it stirs emotions and creativity throughout the business. New organizational structures encourage a degree of conflict and constructively channel the resulting energies that emerge from the resistance to change. Encouraged conflict has to be managed by the leader. Conflict management may be one of the most difficult tasks imposed on the leader; it certainly requires the constant monitoring and immediate attention of leaders.

Conflict can be intra-personal, interpersonal, intra-group and inter-group. Causes of conflict include: role conflict, change in delegation, change in status, change in goals, resource competition and culture conflict. The result of conflicts can be negative (resulting in people not wanting to work together) or can be managed by the leader to create growth opportunities and vitality for the organization.

Conflict avoidance is no longer the norm in the business world, including health care facilities. New rules embrace the concept of conflict and encourage development of conflict management skills. Daily conflict is not only allowed but appropriate levels of conflict are encouraged by top management. Somerville and Mills (1999) believe that the resolution of conflict begins with employees embracing shared values that drive behavior. This allows isolated controversies to rapidly proceed to conflict resolution enabling employees to get back to accomplishing organizational goals.

Followership

In recent years researchers have begun to appreciate the value of true followership for the leader. There is no such thing as a leader without followers. In fact, most of the research involving leaders' traits and qualities supports the belief that the leaders vision must be embraced by followers. Creating a shared vision is one of the imperatives of transformational leadership. A correspondence of positive qualities between leader and followers allows everyone in the organization to experience personal growth by working together for the common good. A follower cannot be separated from the leader in terms of dedication and commitment to organization goals. The only way for leaders to achieve institutional goals is for employees to commit to following the leader. This is where the leader must exhibit required expertise and articulate a message that loyal followers want to hear.

There must also be a match between leaders and followers regarding the vision of what can be accomplished by the business. There must be chemistry between the leaders' will and the followers' ability and effort to complete the various tasks necessary for goal accomplishment. Followers want leaders to be competent, honest, and available, i.e. trustworthy. In order to assure followers that these qualities are present, leaders must demonstrate strong interpersonal skills. In other words, communication becomes a prerequisite to build trust in the leader and faith in his or her vision.

Followership is developed by matching personal goals of employees with the goals of the leaders and the business. It is interesting to note that this type of match most often occurs in a sole proprietorship under the constant attention of a motivated entrepreneur. The entrepreneur has no problem helping followers meet their personal goals as long as his or her vision for the company is becoming reality. Unfortunately, this matching of goals by leaders and followers often erodes as the company grows. The secret to perpetuating motivated growth and vitality lies in finding a way to keep the vision alive even after transition through growth has occurred.

For some, change will mean crisis. For those who are prepared, change offers great opportunities for advancement. Innovation and creativity are the prerequisite for success in the exploitation of the changing health care environment. The leader has the responsibility to create the antecedent conditions necessary to foster the process of creativity.

New research has found that the best followers are independent and critical thinking individuals who are usually creative and innovative. The problem for business is that if these superior followers are not allowed to practice these skills they usually leave the company. Once they leave, they either migrate to competing firms or become entrepreneurs who compete with their former employer. Unfortunately, many administrators attempt to constrain innovation and creativity because they fear loss of power as change occurs and competence is developed and recognized at diversified levels apart from their personal administrative domains. Traditional administrators block innovation through excessive bureaucratic involvement, increasing management isolation, and inappropriate application of incentives.

9

Top management in health care facilities quite often isolates itself because of tremendous fear of confronting loss of bureaucratically granted power and people issues. The current nursing shortage and dissatisfaction in this country speaks to management failure in health care facilities.

It is not possible for followers to commit to administrators who have isolated themselves from the employee base. In such a setting, employees recognize that they are expendable, so they prepare themselves to leave as early in their tenure as possible. They do this by taking advantage of educational programs in preparation for the eventual pink slip. The problem is that they take both their newly acquired skills and their knowledge about their current employer to the competition. The expendable employee understands the need to grow his or her human capital. Unfortunately, the bureaucratic manager underestimates the value of human capital to the organization; or, understanding its value fears that the emergence of expertise among followers will erode his or her power base.

Organizational power is nothing more than the ability to influence others to achieve desired goals. This ability to influence others is found not only in the formally recognized institutional leadership, but it is also found among informal leaders who constantly interact with other followers. A manager is always worrying about losing power and not being in charge. A leader, on the other hand, treats employees as family, enjoys watching them develop and grow, and celebrates their successes. Followers develop trust in the leader and actually thank the leader for the opportunity to offer excellent service to their customers. A leader recognizes that without exemplary followers goal achievement is usually marginal. A leader also understands that through trust followers will help create a thick positive culture committed to goal accomplishment.

The leader is capable of creating conditions in the company that allow followers to experience the empowerment of freedom to innovate. Empowered followers become capable of performing superior feats that surprise both follower and leader. This personal and professional growth experience becomes addictive. In this transactional work environment, the leader just needs to watch employees grow and occasionally clear roadblocks to success.

Many successful companies require future leaders to first be successful followers. In other words, prior to assuming a leadership role in a company one must successfully pass a followership component of development. This allows the future leader to more fully understand the role of employee empowerment and the value of personal growth for all employees.

There are changing patterns in many occupational groups that demand continuous and increasing levels of training and education. This investment in human capital development (training and education) is the property of the employee and not of the company that pays the up front costs. This implies that the educated worker can take the newly developed skills to the highest bidder. This is a major concern of the employer when dealing with knowledgeable workers. Nowhere is this better demonstrated than in the current and projected nursing shortage, especially in long-term care institutions, where the shortage has evolved to crisis proportions. This situation emphasizes the need for leadership in order that the costs incurred in human capital development are recovered through increased productivity of a committed workforce.

Knowledge-based jobs also demand a change in the way we evaluate processes in the production of health care services. In fact, most consumers evaluating health services place a heavier emphasis on how these services are provided rather than on what is produced. Hammer (1996) argues that in order to survive and grow in today's competitive environment, companies must refocus and reorganize themselves around their processes. Institutions must discover what they are capable of doing well and improve upon those areas. Conversely, they must discontinue what they are not able to do well. This allows leadership to allocate limited resources to areas most likely to enhance service to mission. This reorganization of resource allocation will mean that change will impact everyone working in your organization.

Somerville and Mills (1999) argue that the desire to create success for others is the mentality that establishes true leadership. Hammer (1996) also revealed that revolutions usually begin with an attempt at improving the organization that will eventually be brought down by internal forces. Inwardly focused hierarchies do not respond well to fast-paced change. Managers are so busy protecting individual power bases that the organization as a whole proceeds very cautiously with respect to the unknown and quite frequently misses opportunities for growth. During times of rapid change, winning institutions often rely on unconventional approaches geared to exploit change, converting potential threats into real opportunities.

The transformational leader becomes a winner through the creation and sharing of win-win scenarios throughout the organization. Workers who feel the connection with others in the workplace willingly commit the discretionary efforts necessary for extraordinary success.

11

Motivation and Empowerment of Employees

Motivation results from a desire to satisfy unmet needs. It consists of internal and external forces that energize movement toward goal achievement. Unmet needs, the perceived gap between what one has and what one wants, produce an inner tension to create a better future. Employees seek to relieve the tension produced by unmet needs. The employee seeks need satisfaction which can translate into increased productivity if these needs are being satisfied through participation in the workplace. This requires leaders to recognize what factors motivate employees and offer these as incentives to and rewards for increased productivity in the workplace.

Daft (2001) found that rewards might be intrinsic or extrinsic, system-wide or individual. Intrinsic rewards represent internal satisfactions enjoyed by the worker for performing certain tasks. Extrinsic rewards are supplied to the worker by another individual, usually a supervisor or leader. System-wide rewards apply to all employees in the organization, while individual rewards are different for each employee. Taken together, these rewards energize and sustain workers, allowing personal growth and allowing their institution to become a truly excellent company.

Motivation is an important component of excellence in the delivery of services. For health care institutions a motivational environment allows attraction of the best employees, retention of the best employees, and promotion of good citizenship behaviors among employees. Good citizenship is reflected in employees' willingness to speak well of their company when they are not at work. This behavior allows the health care facility to attract more loyal employees and customers. Such commitment to the company cannot be purchased or coerced; it must be earned by trustworthy leadership.

Most organizational researchers believe that motivation works best when it is based on self-governance. Employees usually begin their tenures as motivated workers, but as time passes they lose the impulse to strive for excellence. The leader needs to find the triggers that motivate the majority of employees and nurture a workplace environment that supplies these factors. This task can become almost a full-time activity for the leader, but it is time well spent.

The main financial concern for health care facilities in the foreseeable future is the progressively difficult task of increasing productivity in the delivery of health services. If productivity is to be increased there needs to be a focus on adding value to services. This will require improved performance by all members of the organization. Two requirements for increased performance are employee ability and employee effort. Ability represents human capital that must be nurtured and respected. Effort is best determined by motivation, and enhanced effort requires workforce desire and commitment. These requirements for improved productivity are usually found in the small companies run by entrepreneurs.

Poor or substandard productivity in any business requires that leadership determine if the cause is lack of ability, lack of motivation, or both. If it is determined to be lack of ability, an appropriate training program may solve the problem. If the problem is lack of motivation, the leader must strike a principled deal with employees where an exchange is negotiated involving satisfying employee goals in return for desired employee action. If the problem is both, then leadership of the organization has failed.

An entrepreneur is probably the most motivated worker in the country. He or she has no starting or quitting time for work and never stops thinking about the business. These are the types of individuals that health care facilities definitely need if they are to survive, grow and prosper. These motivated individuals take risks, sometimes with tremendous success, because they are truly empowered. The business is theirs; they own it.

Kuratko and Welsch (2001) found it is important for the leader to keep an entrepreneurial frame of mind in order to avoid regressing to a bureaucratic mind-set and stifling innovation. Entrepreneurship is the act of forming new organizations while intra-preneurship is the act of creating new products and services within larger organizations. Intra-preneurship occurs within the company and is an achievement of motivated employees. Quite often the act of intra-preneurship requires little more than a change in the process of delivering services to the customer. Capturing the creative energies and enthusiasm of intrapreneurs will be a challenge and opportunity for health care organizations in the 21st century.

The process of intra-preneurship does not work well in a bureaucracy. The generative energies of intrapreneurs need a more organic empowering organizational structure to achieve success.. Organic organizational structure grants employees broader responsibilities, decentralizes decision-making and encourages risk-taking by all employees.

The challenge to leadership now becomes framed in the question "How do we get this level of motivation and commitment in our followers?" A second question seems to follow: "How do we achieve the practice of good

13

corporate citizenship among the majority of our followers?" The answer is to create small business units within the company and allow employees to take responsibility and be rewarded for a successful venture. This requires the leader to empower subordinates to run their share of the company. The value of true empowerment of the employee for the organization can be enormous. It can allow the employee to satisfy higher level needs and encourage exploration of further higher level need satisfaction through win-win scenarios.

Total Quality Management (TQM)

Empowered, highly motivated employees are able to rise to a higher level of service to consumers. This involves becoming the best and then competing with yourself to become even better. It offers every employee the opportunity for continuous personal and professional growth. As the employee grows, the health care facility prospers.

The leadership methodology best suited to fostering such growth processes is Total Quality Management (TQM). Properly committed to by leadership, TQM behaves like a computer virus by infecting every part of the organization. Healthy competition to become the best and then to become even better is the only way to guarantee continuous improvement in the organization.

TQM has been around since before World War II in the business world and more recently has been introduced to the delivery of health care services. Berwick, Godfrey & Roessner (1999), define TQM and emphasize its focus on the processes of health care delivery. Understanding process allows employees to play the role of customer (receiving work from others), processor (adding value) and supplier (giving work to others). The process of adding value is most important because the customer is the arbiter of quality. The customer decides what constitutes added value. In order for value to be added and in order to foster continuous quality improvement, every member of the health care facility must maintain a customer focus, understanding that both internal customers as well as ultimate consumers of health care must be satisfied.

Health care facilities are beginning to be evaluated on the basis of outcomes. Achievement of valued outcomes will influence the way we design health care organizations. Valid and precise outcome measurements are crucial to the future success of the organization. The process changes resulting from the environmental, technological, demographic and reimbursement challenges, as well as in the structure and function of the health care organization as a whole requires organizational redesign.

A major cause of transformation in organizational design is environmental change. If the environment changes it stands to reason that the way we deliver services to customers will also change. The new health care facility must become obsessed with quality and focus on the demands of increasingly informed consumers.

The Learning Organization

In the past the health care industry existed in a relatively sheltered and stable environment and therefore traditional management styles and bureaucracy worked well. Plans could be developed and managers could usually achieve goals with little need for innovation or transformational leadership. This bureaucratic structure not only resisted change but also wanted nothing to do with change agents. That idyllic landscape all changed with the realization that even health care would be forced to cope with limited resources amid rising consumer expectations. Something had to replace traditional bureaucratic managerial processes. Now the need for change is a daily quest demanding maverick leaders and committed followers.

The demise of the adequacy of traditional management behaviors has ushered in the concept of the learning organization. Descriptions of and theories supporting the learning organization have achieved chapter status in most new books about management and leadership. But what is a learning organization and why should the concept be of concern to health care facilities?

Daft (2001) describes the learning organization as one that involves everyone in the identification and solution of problems. The learning organization is based on equality, elimination of hierarchy, and a shared positive culture. All employees, in effect, become leaders and mentors because of their special areas of expertise.

A majority of individuals appear to believe that the receipt of one's final diploma marks the end of the formal learning process. In the past this belief may very well have been functional because it took a long time for knowledge to be gathered, analyzed and then disseminated to others. Technology has made new information available to everyone almost concurrent with its discovery. All that is required is the knowledge of where information is housed and how to access it. Continuous learning has become the most important component of future organizational success.

15

Learning usually consists of acquiring knowledge and experiences. While a single individual is severely limited in the amount of learning he or she can absorb at any given time, a team of followers has almost unlimited potential to attain new knowledge to assist in the continuous improvement of the process of service delivery. Great leaders are usually both great teachers and great learners. These leaders work to create a learning environment throughout the company that becomes a means of rapidly disseminating new knowledge and experiences to all employees, allowing everyone to achieve both personal and professional growth on a daily basis. The learning organization compels everyone to join in the experience of developing new skills to deal with the ever-present process of rapid change.

Gouillart and Kelly (1999) argue that a firm must invest in its employees first and worry about productivity increases and profit later. It is like the investment in a certificate of deposit where you invest your money up front and receive the rewards at a future time. Employees must be looked at as human beings with enormous potential if allowed to develop. By developing the human capital of the firm, leaders are providing growth in the most essential asset that the organization can make available in furtherance of mission.

NOTES:

NOTES:

18

CHAPTER 2

Quality Issues in Health Care Delivery

By: Thomas Ross, Ph.D.
Assistant Professor of Health Care Administration
King's College

Introduction

A board member should be an advocate for the community in which the hospital or health system is located. The paramount responsibility of hospital boards is to oversee the operations of the organization including its management, financial status and the quality of health care delivered. This chapter provides a framework for evaluating the quality of health care provided, ties quality to the health care delivery process and discusses the potential impact of quality programs on the financial performance of the organization.

A generic definition of quality is the degree to which a good or service meets established standards or satisfies the customer. This definition recognizes the two dimensions of quality. First is the technical definition, meeting established standards. Organizations such as GE and Motorola use the six-sigma approach that establishes a goal of 3.4 product failures for every 1,000,000 products produced. Errors in health care resulting in death or injury to patients are receiving increased scrutiny, the Institute of Medicine (2000) reports that up to 98,000 patients are killed each year due to medical errors – obviously medicine has a long way to travel before it reaches the six-sigma threshold.

The second dimension is not concerned with reaching technical standards but rather asks the simple question "does the good or service satisfy the consumer?" Argument often arises over the "correct" definition of quality but it is clear that goods or products that meet technical standards but fail to satisfy customers will fail to attract business and drain resources from an organization. Beta video recording machines are a recent example of a product that was touted to be superior to VHS machines but failed to generate consumer loyalty. On the other hand, customers may be delighted with a good or service but if the product does not meet expectations the organization and its employees are unlikely to be satisfied with their performance and huge liability claims may eventually arise. Quality health care must meet technical standards and the expectations of patients.

19

Quality in health care can be defined as appropriate care from qualified providers delivered in the in the most appropriate manner and setting for the patient's unique circumstances. This definition emphasizes that the services rendered to the patient must first be necessary and effective. Second, the right provider should deliver the care – this should be the lowest cost provider who can capably do the work. High quality is not achieved by using highly skilled and highly paid personnel to perform tasks that can be accomplished by lower paid individuals. Conversely, lower paid personnel cannot be employed for tasks for which they are not qualified. Quality care requires the right person for the right job. Third, care should be delivered competently with consideration of the patient's expectations. This requires effective performance that meets the patient's desires for courtesy and respect. Fourth, care should be delivered in the correct setting. We do not want to see services that can be provided in a physician's office delivered in the ER or have a patient hospitalized when home health services or nursing home care can be used. Finally, we do not want to apply a one-size fits all solution to every patient but rather design treatment plans to the particular medical needs of each patient.

How do we design and monitor a quality management program to accomplish all these objectives when multiple different providers deliver health care services on a patient-by-patient basis? First we must define what we mean by quality, that is, what are we going to measure? An interesting approach is the five Ds of quality. The five D's: death, disability, disease, discomfort and dissatisfaction succinctly identify the primary concerns of patients and providers. Death refers to mortality rates, disability to the minimization or absence of impairment arising from disease or injury, disease to the successful eradication of the condition that the patient presented with, discomfort to the minimization or absence of pain during and after treatment of a disease or injury and dissatisfaction to patient's happiness with and approval of the care received. This categorization scheme demonstrates that quality measurement must be undertaken in multiple dimensions and that programs that focus on one or two components will miss the majority of the picture.

A quality management program must be designed around the idea of ensuring optimal care across a continuum of care provided by multiple providers. Eddy (1990a) notes that quality health care is determined by the decisions establishing the treatment plan and the execution of the plan. The rest of this chapter examines practice policies as a tool of quality management and how they affect medical decision-making, how to structure a quality management system and the potential impact of quality programs on the organization's financial performance.

Medical Decision-Making

Securing the support of practitioners is the biggest obstacle faced by those attempting to implement quality management programs. Health care has always been characterized by physician autonomy; quality management and calls for increased accountability are often viewed as striking at this autonomy. The health care industry has been known for hopping on to the latest management fads be it management by objectives, total quality management or continuous quality improvement. The poor track records of these initiatives puts additional pressure on new programs because credibility is often absent and busy practitioners do not want to invest in activities that may be discarded in the near future. If quality management programs are to succeed, practitioners must be involved in goal setting, be confident in the practices implemented and believe that the benefits of the program will exceed their costs.

Ensuring quality health care will require the creation and monitoring of practice policies. That is we must have a firm idea of what services should be rendered to a patient, the ability to recognize when appropriate and inappropriate deviations from these treatment plans. In some cases these policies will prescribe what tests and procedures should be performed on an hour-by-hour basis for each day of an inpatient admission. Anyone can sympathize with physicians who have invested in extensive training for their profession to be wary of being reduced to following prefabricated treatment plans. Many physicians fear that practice policies will lead to reductions in their professional autonomy and clinical judgment and pursue cost reduction over quality improvement. Understandable as these fears are they arise from a lack of understanding of practice policies.

Clearly stating the case for practice policies, defining and differentiating the different types of practice policies and establishing when each will be used should reduce practitioner fears. Practice policies range from standards to guidelines to options. Each is built upon substantially different assumptions concerning physician and patient understanding of treatment choices and outcomes. Understanding each policy type is vital to avoiding unnecessary conflict, building consensus and achieving goals.

A practice standard as defined by Nash (1999) is a value or criterion established by authority, custom or general consent as a model or example to guide performance and to measure quantity or quality. Standards define correct medical practice. Standards describe practices with documented outcomes and virtual unanimity among patients about the desirability of the treatment (James, (1993)). When standards exists they should be applied

21

rigidly, that is followed in all cases (Eddy, (1990d)). When practice deviates from standards it is essential that the quality management personnel identify why the deviation occurred, determine if the deviation was appropriate based on the unique circumstances of the patient or resulted from a lack of familiarity with good medical practice. These definitions recognize the practice standard as the benchmark against which patient care must be judged. Using more or less medical services than necessary is poor quality and represents an opportunity to educate practitioners and improve outcomes.

Medical services can be under-used, over-used or misused. Under-use occurs when services that could improve health outcomes are not delivered. Over-use occurs when services are rendered where the benefits of the intervention are less than the treatment risks i.e. procedural risks, anesthetic risks and/or iatrogenic effects. Misuse occurs when the appropriate care is poorly delivered. Practice policies are one means to attempt to control these types of errors and hospitals should implement procedures to ensure that standards are followed. Fear of standards and assuming all practice policies will be rigid standards often produces the derisive and dismissive comments of "cookbook medicine" from practitioners.

Practice guidelines are a less strict form of practice policy that recognize the non-deterministic nature of medical practice and need for professional discretion. Practice guidelines according to Nash (1999) are a scientifically determined set of specifications for the provision of care in given disease or injury categories. James (1993) defines guidelines as clinical interventions with documented outcomes but whose outcomes are not clear desirable to all patients. Eddy (1990d) sees guidelines as flexible reference points that should be followed in most cases. The role of the hospital should be to make sure that physicians are aware of the appropriate treatment options, monitor patient care to insure these options are used and disseminate information on the outcomes and costs of each approach to practitioners.

Options are clinical interventions for which outcomes are not known or where different patients may prefer divergent treatment plans (James (1993)). Eddy (1990d) notes options are neutral with respect to recommending an intervention. An option is simply one of many acceptable treatment interventions where interaction between the physician and patient (or the patient's advocate) should determine the treatment approach pursued. When multiple treatment plans can be used the hospital should monitor the different clinical outcomes, patient satisfaction and costs of each options and present this information to practitioners.

Figure 2.1 demonstrates the impact of practice policies on physician discretion as we move from standards to options.

Figure 2.1 – Practice Policies and Physician Discretion

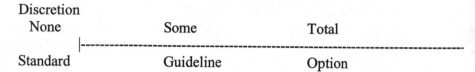

Will quality health care require standardization and limits on autonomy or will physicians continue to exercise their professional judgment with options providing minimal guidance? Recognizing the difference between standards, guidelines and options and when each should be used is essential to assessing the impact on physician discretion. The use of standards, guidelines and options and where health care will operate on this continuum will be determined by patient preferences and clinical effectiveness.

Patient Preferences

Today's medical literature abounds with articles on how to incorporate patient preferences into medical decision-making. The days of paternalistic decision-making in medicine are waning. Paternalism in medicine as noted by Charles et al (1999) relied on four critical assumptions, the first is for most illnesses there is a single optimal treatment and most physicians are familiar with the treatment. The other three assumptions are: physicians will consistently select optimal treatments, because of physician's information advantage they are in the best position to evaluate treatment trade-offs and make care decisions, and their concern for patient welfare is sufficient inducement to ensure correct treatments are selected. These assumptions are erroneous. Patients are less willing to uncritically accept physician recommendations and are using emerging information technologies to become knowledgeable about their condition in order to assume an integral role in deciding their treatment plan.

Rising consumerism makes it imperative that patients not only receive an explanation of what treatments are contemplated and the possible outcomes but also be offered an active role in selecting treatment plans when guidelines and options exist that produce different outcomes or side effects. In these cases the patient should be given the opportunity to actively participate in the decision-making process so their values are incorporated into the treatment plan. Lutz and Shaman (2001) add two additional implications of health care consumerism, the first is that providers must develop innovative services to meet patient's desires for choice, convenience and easy assess. Second, providers must streamline processes to respond to consumer demands for lower costs and prices.

Besides cultivating patient goodwill, legal precedents are pushing providers to supply more information to patients and be more responsive to their preferences. *Canterbury v Spence* in 1972 was a landmark case that established the right of informed consent and imposed on providers the obligation to inform patients of all the information that a reasonable patient should know. This required providers to explain to patients the potential risks and benefits of a proposed treatment prior to delivery of care. *In re Quinlan* the court found a patient's right to decide their end of life treatment i.e. a right to decline treatment. The right to decline treatment was upheld in *Cruzan v Director Mo. Dept of Health* but the court demanded that clear and convincing evidence of the patient's wishes exist prior to discontinuation of treatment. These cases expanded patient's rights in the areas of informed consent and participation in treatment decisions and established documentation standards required to prove a patient's intentions prior to implementing their treatment preferences.

When should a patient's preferences be incorporated into the medical decision-making process? Owen (1998) holds that they should be incorporated when disease or treatment affects the quality of life or when treatment involves risk or side effects that could impact length of life. Eddy (1990a) specifies three treatment principles to incorporate patient preferences into medical decisions. First, decisions should be based on outcomes that are important to patients. Is the quality or quantity of life most important to the patient? Second, the physician is responsible for estimating the effects of treatment on outcomes as accurately as possible given available evidence and conveying this information to the patient. Finally, the preferences assigned to each outcome should reflect patient's preferences. The physician should not impose his values on the patient but allow the values of the patient to prevail.

Everyone knows someone whose divergent values led him or her to undergo a treatment or forego care where if we were placed in the same situation we would decide the other way. Perhaps the most extreme and illustrative case of divergent preferences lies with Do Not Resuscitate orders. John Coombs (1999) during a seminar on quality management reported that physicians were only able to accurately assess 6.25 percent of the time a patient's preference for resuscitation and 40 percent of patients did not want to discuss the issue. This example illustrates the difficulty of eliciting and knowing another's preference for care in a truly life or death situation.

24

Why do preferences for medical care vary? People place different values on life and health, have divergent beliefs about the health care industry and the effectiveness of medical treatments, and vary in their ability to assess their condition, their need for care or the potential treatment risks. These differences manifest themselves in the multitude of treatment plans utilized to treat a single condition. Multiple studies have attempted to discover if patient preferences vary systematically with patient demographic characteristics.

Stiggelbout and Kiebert (1997) found that older patients and men take a more passive role in medical decision-making. Patients, relative to their companions who accompanied them to medical services, were more passive regarding treatment decisions. Stigglebout and Kiebert attribute this passivity to the effect of sickness and recommends that physicians be more active in encouraging sick patients to participate in the decision-making process. Karlson et al (1997) in another study on the effects of gender differences found men chose surgery earlier and had higher expectations of success. Women were more likely to accept pain and attempt to avoid surgery to minimize disruptions to their usual lifestyle. They conclude that differences in medical utilization are not attributable to differential physician advice but arose from different gender preferences.

The expectations of the success of a medical treatment should influence the desirability of medical treatment but what determines these expectations? Patient satisfaction will be heavily influenced by how well treatment meets their expectations. Kravitz et al (1996) studied unmet patient expectations and found that they were determined by their somatic symptoms, vulnerability, past experience and transmitted knowledge. Somatic symptoms include functional impairment, duration of symptoms, intensity and seriousness, of these duration and intensity of symptoms were the dominant factors. A patient's vulnerability was measured by his or her age, family history, lifestyle and prior illness. Reducing unmet expectations require physicians to recognize these factors and incorporate them into their treatment plan. They found one of the largest sources of unmet expectations were the pronouncements of other clinicians only duration of symptoms was more important. In their conclusion, simple "demand management" schemes are discounted given the complex relationships they found but the fact that dissatisfaction arises from the different clinical information of different clinicians speaks to the need for more consistency in the health care delivery process to increase patient satisfaction.

Schecter et al (1996) in a study of cardiac catherization found the patients with less education, those with poor cardiac function, no previous catherization or from a non-referral community hospital and smokers were more likely to disagree with cardiac catherization. No difference was detected between women and men's preference for or receipt of cardiac catherization. This study is significant because it highlights the need for physicians to convey to patients some minimal information regarding their condition and treatment and cultivate their reasoning ability.

Shelbourne, Strum and Wells (1999) take issue with the emphasis on clinical issues and undertook a study to determine what role mental and social issues play in determining patient preferences. They found that mental and social health issues were almost as important as physical issues in determining patient preferences. Social health was defined as the ability to develop, maintain and nurture major social relationships. Studies show that physicians are concerned with disease specific clinical syndromes and less sensitive to morbidity, pain and suffering which are the primary concerns of patients. The authors suggest that by concentrating on clinical issues physicians overlook and devalue the effect of treatments on a patient's ability to maintain important social relationships.

How do preferences for medical care vary? Coley et al (1996) found that 74 percent of patients with pneumonia preferred home care to hospitalization. Of those surveyed 69 percent stated their physician was solely responsible for determining the location of care and only 11 percent were asked for their preference. Patients in this case not only considered home care a higher value but home care also carries with it the secondary benefit of lower cost. Weeks et al (1998) found that patient preferences for life-extending therapies with toxic effects versus comfort care were determined by prognosis. Patients expecting to live at least six months desired life-extending treatments. As stated earlier men and women were found to have different preferences for surgery and this difference was not attributed to differential physician advice. These findings demonstrated the divergence in patient preference for different types of intervention and the responsibility of physicians to understand patient values prior to establishing treatment plans.

How should physicians incorporate patient's preferences into health care decisions? First the physician must determine if the patient wants to participate in the decision-making process and if so, to what extent. Eddy (1990a) describes the medical decision process in five components. The primary input is evidence, what outcomes have been produced by certain interventions for a given condition? The second component requires the physician to use his or her judgment to analyze the available evidence to determine what the likely outcome for alternative interventions will be for his or her patient. Given the probable outcomes, what decision would the

26

patient take if they had complete information? At this point the physician must determine the patient's preferences and incorporate them into the medical decision-making process to decide what treatments should be undertaken. Figure 2.2 diagrams this process.

Figure 2.2 – Steps in Medical Decision-Making

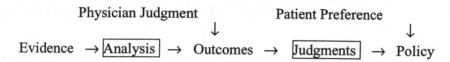

Eddy's diagram illustrates his contention that errors in the decision-making process arise from misperceptions of outcomes or preferences. To improve health care it is essential that the system is designed to provide physicians with easier access to medical literature to inform their analysis and explicit processes be developed to incorporate patient preferences into the deliberation over treatment options.

Eddy (1990b) provides a seven-step process to improve medical decision-making, table 2.1. The first five steps depend on the physician's ability to locate and evaluate medical information. As daunting as this task is, the incorporation of patient preferences in step 6 may present the bigger challenge. The difficulty arises from attempting to reconcile the different worldviews of professionals trained in the scientific method and the often-unsubstantiated values, beliefs and biases of patients. If the evidence and preferences can be identified, step 7 is a simple task of selecting a treatment plan that produces the best medical outcome while honoring the patient's preferences.

Table 2.1 – A Medical Decision-Making Process

1. Identify treatment options.
2. Identify outcomes of each option.
3. Evaluate evidence pertaining to each outcome.
4. Estimate consequences of each option.
5. Weigh trade-offs.
6. Factor in patient preferences.
7. Select an option.

Using this decision-making process on a patient-by-patient basis is impossible and would be undesirable even if it were possible. Physicians do not have the time nor does society want to invest the resources to make such a process work. Practice policies are needed to simplify the process. Practice policies establish templates that streamline decision-making and treatment allowing physicians to concentrate their expertise on those cases where policies should not be applied.

Will the benefits of including patient preferences in treatment decisions be greater than the effort and cost? Trends in health care indicate that patients and their families expect to be actively involved in the decision-making process and that the resulting medical decisions reflect their preferences. Patients assign higher value to treatments that reflect their preferences. We can expect that patient satisfaction will increase with their involvement in the decision-making process and the treatment plans that result. Practitioners should benefit from greater patient buy-in to treatment plans and greater patient compliance with orders. Provider satisfaction should increase as better care processes and outcomes are achieved. Jensen (1999) argues that a larger role for patients in the decision-making process will also result in greater patient acceptance of poor outcomes. Finally, society should see an increase in health care effectiveness that could reduce the need for remedial care and reduce health care spending.

Research on patient preferences is clear that patients have very different ideas on what treatment options are most desirable and their preferences cannot easily be deduced through socio-economic characteristics. Patients and physicians do not view the world through the same lens; patients are concerned with morbidity, pain and suffering while physicians are more concerned with disease specific clinical syndromes. This difference emphasizes the need to evaluate treatment plans from the patient's perspective as well as from a clinical effectiveness perspective. In terms of our discussion of practice policies the use of guidelines and options over standards is clearly indicated given the disparity of patient preferences. In the words of Vickery and Lynch (1997) "Understanding the perceptions, attitudes, and beliefs that determine patient behavior is essential to improving health care."

Evidence Based Medicine

Patients will seldom be able to compete with the breath of medical knowledge and experience held by practitioners so evaluating the effectiveness of treatment is clearly the duty of the physician. However, many are critical of medicine's track record on the use of evidence. Those who think that medicine has often lacked scientific rigor are leading the evidence based medicine movement. According to the Evidence Based Medicine Working Group (1992) evidence based medicine "de-emphasizes intuition, unsystematic clinical experience, and pathophysiologic rationale as

28

sufficient grounds for clinical decision making and stresses the examination of evidence from clinical research."

Brent James (1993) notes that between 80-90 percent of medical practice is unfounded. This does not mean that 80-90 percent of medical practice is ineffective or inefficient but that it evolved over time and was not founded on clinical studies. The drawbacks of the traditional approach, that is "standard and accepted" practice, are its circular reasoning foundation, what people should do (policies) is what people are doing (standard practice), and its reliance on subjective decision-making (Eddy (1990c)). The evolved standards of care may be the most effective but we do not know this due to the absence of clinical trials that compare interventions. One of the biggest problems that medicine faces is it decentralization; independent physicians have been able to practice their own style of care. James (1993) notes, "Individual clinicians showed differences in practice patterns from patient to patient. In fact, it appeared that a single clinician sometimes was inconsistent when treating the same patient from day to day, or even from morning to evening rounds."

The sheer diversity in practice styles has made it difficult to determine what the optimal treatment for a condition should be. It is difficult to determine the impact of changing one variable in a treatment plan when there is no constancy in any part of the plan. That is when all other medical services are used in different amounts and combinations how is it possible to determine what improves or reduces health outcomes? Practice policies are needed to establish benchmark processes and outcomes against which different approaches to treatment can be assessed.

Assessing treatments and improving patient care is the purpose of case management. Case management is an outcome driven approach that involves all appropriate health providers in planning the course and direction of care for specific patients. Case management is commonly targeted to high risk and high cost patients. Theoretically the process starts with identifying unexplained clinical variations that is differences in treatment and outcomes that cannot be traced to differences in the patient's condition. Once this variation is identified the institution must determine if standardization is needed and if so, how should it be standardize? Standards can be established through the use of expert opinion, evaluation of clinical research or some combination of each. James (1993) notes that the standard selected is not as important as standardization itself. One has to have a fixed baseline to gauge alterations in a process and hence a local standard will work. He notes that "No matter where a group starts, the iterative application of the scientific

29

method, informed by comparisons with other professional groups, will eventually lead to documented best patient care."

We know patients generally do not have sufficient information to decide what is the appropriate treatment for their condition but how well informed are physicians? Wide differences in practice style and considerable uncertainty over outcomes and effectiveness exist in medicine. John Wennberg and his colleagues documented the wide differences in the use of medical services between populations that were homogeneous. By studying similar populations, they minimize the impact of population differences on medical usage and concentrate on the role of practice style in explaining the different utilization rates.

Concerns over variation in medical use grew after Wennberg and Gittlesohn's path breaking 1973 article. They documented differences in the use of diagnostic x-ray, electrocardiogram and laboratory services of 400 percent, 600 percent and 700 percent in New England. They conclude that differences in utilization were uncorrelated with differences in mortality rates and were positively related to the number of physicians and beds in the community. In a follow-up, Wennberg and Gittlesohn (1982) documented twofold differences in the use of surgery in the six states of New England. Among the most common procedures, hysterectomy, prostatectomy and tonsillectomy, the rate between areas varied by a much as 600 percent. The difference in utilization was again attributed to differences in the number and types of physicians and number of hospital beds not to differences in patient need. In areas with a large number of physicians and hospital beds they found high hospitalization rates. They hypothesize that variations in utilization were highest for those procedures whose benefits and risks were least understood.

In 1989, Wennberg et al studied mortality rates between Boston and New Haven and found that despite using 44 percent more hospital days and spending twice as much per capita, Boston's overall mortality rates were nearly identical to New Haven. It is widely believed that physicians practice patterns are determined by the patterns of their colleagues in a given market and these studies suggest that significant improvement in the health system can be achieved by reconciling the differences in utilization and practice styles.

Given the curious lack of impact of higher utilization and expenditures on outcomes in Wennberg's studies, will practice policies improve care? James (1993) in his work on adult respiratory distress syndrome (ARDS) studied the practical issues surrounding guideline implementation in a hospital.

30

James found that one of the major benefits of the implementation was bringing practitioners together to understand the differences in their practice patterns and providing them objective data to evaluate patient care. After the implementation of practice guidelines, patient survival rates for their high-risk patients averaged 44 percent compared with rates of 9 percent-15 percent for other providers. Improvements in patient outcomes would themselves justify the guideline but in addition the guidelines allowed physicians to reduce the time needed to manage patients, reduce patient time in ICU and lower annual treatment costs.

In a more far-reaching article, Grimshaw and Russell (1993) surveyed 59 clinical guidelines and found that 55 of these studies detected improvements in the process of care and of eleven studies that measured outcomes, nine detected significant improvement in outcomes. Many of these studies also showed significant increases in patient compliance. They conclude that the studies where little or no improvements in health outcomes were demonstrated may be the result of poor implementation of guidelines rather than ineffective guidelines.

Table 2.2 combines patient preferences and outcomes to illustrate when standards, guidelines and options should be used. Three levels of patient preferences are recognized, unanimous, majority and unknown. Unanimous indicates all patients would select the same treatment plan given their condition, values and treatment options. Majority preferences suggest a preponderance of patients would select the same treatment plan given their condition, values and treatment options. Unknown preferences cover a wide range of scenarios. Patients may be indifferent to the available options, there may be significant and distinct populations that prefer one option to another or studies of patient preferences have not been undertaken.

Outcomes are scaled from well documented to indeterminate, well-documented outcomes are those that practitioners generally accept the effectiveness of one option over others. In the middle range is inconclusive indicating that there is no clear superiority of one intervention over another, which could be the result of varying skills of the practitioners i.e. one physician can produce better results with one therapy while another is more capable and can produce a similar outcome with another treatment or superiority depends on other factors. Finally we have indeterminate where evidence is lacking or the evidence is contradictory.

Table 2.2 – Deciding Among Standards, Guidelines and Options

Outcome Preferences	Well Documented Outcomes	Inconclusive Documentation	Indeterminate
Unanimous	Standard	Guideline	Option
Majority	Guideline	Guideline	Option
Unknown/ Indifferent	Option	Option	Option

Table 2.2 clearly shows that fears of intrusions on clinical authority (or cookbook medicine) are unfounded. Only when patient's preferences are known and unanimous and the clinical evidence is strong and well documented would a practice policy (standard) limit a practitioner's judgment. This speaks to the need for practitioners to understand their patients as well as the clinical research that underpins medical practice.

Few would argue that the majority of medicine practice should rely on guidelines and options rather than standards but who can argue that greater scientific rigor will not produce better health outcomes under any practice policy? We clearly need to increase our understanding of medical science and the preferences of patients and incorporate this information into the decision making process. This is an area of great difficulty and contention, where does medical science end and medical art begin? Clinical research needs to address guidelines and options. Population based patient preferences are inadequate to treat individuals when patient preferences are anything other than unanimous. Communication between physicians and patients must increase so physicians can determine their patient's values and incorporate their wishes into the treatment plan.

The push for greater uniformity in medical practice is propelled by four major factors. The first is financial pressure, since the inception of the Prospective Payment System in 1983 and continuing through the Balanced Budget Act of 1997 hospitals found themselves under greater financial pressure. Reduced revenues have led them to explore ways of reducing costs by focusing on valuing adding services and eliminating superfluous, unnecessary services. Hence it is essential to understand what services should be provided and how these services affect patient outcomes.

A second factor is the spread of technology. Technology encompasses two areas: medical care technology and information system technology. The rapid advance of medical technology requires health care providers to determine when new technologies should be adopted. Do these technologies produce superior outcomes relative to existing methods? Answering this

32

question requires us to have a baseline process and outcome to gauge the new technology against. Information technologies provide greater ability to track current health care processes and outcomes and compare these processes against the emerging medical technologies. Besides the improvement in performance and lower cost of hardware and software, there is a concomitant increase in computer literacy and drive for standardization of medical terminology. These trends are going to provide the tools and personnel needed to determine which treatments produce the best clinical outcomes and greatest patient satisfaction.

Clinicians and patients are both concerned over inappropriate care. Shekelle et al (1998) examined over-utilization of medical services for coronary revascularization and hysterectomy and under-use of coronary revascularization. The rates of over-utilization ranged from 3.8 percent to 7.3 percent for coronary revascularization and 31.4 percent to 52.0 percent for hysterectomy. The percentage of patients that should have received coronary revascularization but did not ranged from 31.1 percent to 38.5 percent. Becher and Chassin (2001) report that 24 million Americans inappropriately received antibiotics for colds and viral infections in 1992. They also found that 16 percent of hysterectomies and 23 percent of tympanostomies had inadequate clinical justification. On the under-use side, they found that only 55 percent of patient with atrial fibrillation received anticoagulation to reduce the risk of stroke. These studies illustrate a few of the examples of how patients are exposed to unnecessary treatment risks and often do not receive necessary care. Inappropriate care, either over-use or under-use, has a significant impact on health care expenditures. When over-use occurs, society wastes resources on unnecessary care and additional costs are incurred dealing with complications of treatment. When necessary services are not provided society will incur higher costs whenever the cost of prevention is less than the cure, as noted above treating a stroke patient is more costly than proactive administration of coagulation.

The rapid increase in health care costs and frequent reports of poor outcomes has stimulated the drive for improving health care quality and increasing accountability. Government, employers, insurers and patients have all leapt into the fray. These groups are beginning to demand that they receive demonstrable value for their health dollars. The challenge to health care professionals is to demonstrate to these groups that the services they produce are effective and efficient, we cannot expect society to continue to fund health care while ignoring its demands for accountability. Physicians need to embrace practice policies and quality management programs to insure that they guide their development, implementation and use.

33

Despite societal pressures for change, significant obstacles impede the drive to standardize and rationalize the practice of medicine. Much of the resistance to practice policies is due to misunderstanding of their goals and potential impact on medical decision-making. Physicians are accustomed to autonomous decision-making so any programs that threaten their autonomy are certain to produce resistance. This independence is ingrained into physicians by their collective history, their training and their work experience. It is vital that quality management programs be placed under the direction of the medical staff. The hospital's role in this process should be providing practitioners with the understanding and tools to manage their practices. Hospital administrators must remember that they need to control the health care delivery process not the health care providers.

It is the fear of control and performance assessment that must be overcome. Physicians are leery of being evaluated by non-medical personnel and in this day and age when hospitals are divesting themselves of physicians and managed care organizations are choosing not to renew contracts with physicians, it is essential that quality assessment not be interpreted as a way to get rid of high cost physicians or place blame. These programs must be seen as a means of improving patient care and keeping practitioners abreast of changing medical practice. Siegel et al (1990) report that information is doubling every 10 to 15 years and that there are 20,000 medical journals and 17,000 medical books published annually. Quality management and performance assessment should be seen as one method of keeping physicians abreast of a literature that is expanding beyond the ability of any single individual to read and understand.

A real problem of evidence exists, not only is it voluminous and expanding it is often difficult to obtain and contradictory. Health care practitioners can cite contrary studies for a multitude of conditions and assert that they are too busy providing care to read every journal article published. A major role for the institution is to facilitate access to medical literature, support the creation of standards, guidelines and options by practitioners, and monitor these policies once established. A major concern of physicians is time, how much time does it take them to locate information and once it is obtained will it enable them to see more patients. By providing access to information, practice policies and monitoring hospitals can reduce the administrative aspects of medical practice and increase the amount of time practitioners can allocate to patients. No one wants to dictate treatment plans to physicians but it is clear that quality and accountability issues will require greater standardization and oversight of medical care.

Structuring a Quality Management Program

High quality health care must meet technical standards and satisfy patients. The quality management system constructed must be explicit about what the goals of the program are, what factors will be measured to assess performance, who is responsible for goal setting, monitoring and corrective action, and the process and tools to be used for data collection, management and reporting.

Practice policies should be an integral part of the quality program; these policies present the expected technical standards. They specify who should receive care, who should deliver care, what services should be given, when and how the services should be rendered and where the services should be performed. A comprehensive quality management system must be able to measure compliance with each criterion.

The goal of providing optimal care must be the primary focus of any quality management program. Patients want to be assured that they are receiving the best treatment and employees want to take pride in providing that care. Quality programs flounder when the goal is seen as pointless measurement or cost containment. Clear and generally accepted outcome measures must be selected that leave no doubt that optimal patient care is the goal. To establish credibility and debunk the idea that the program is a bureaucratic exercise, redesign of medical practices and improvements in patient outcomes must be demonstrated.

Does redesigning medical practice mean that the number of services rendered and their cost will increase, decrease or remain the same? Improving health outcomes will produce each of these results depending on the type of medical care we focus our attention on. The goal of quality management when applied to technical standards is to reduce the variance in services provided. That is it should establish guidelines regarding appropriate patient care that ensure that over or under-use of services does not occur. Wide deviation in practice patterns for a single medical condition is assumed to indicate poor care, some patients are subjected to too many tests and procedures while others are under-served.

The issue is not as complex for patient satisfaction. The goal is to increase patient satisfaction and reduce the variance in satisfaction ratings. We want more satisfied patients to ensure their continued patronage and consistently high ratings i.e. we do not want a high average with a wide variance because that indicates we please the majority of our patients but there is a significant subset of patients that are unhappy and unlikely to return.

Support of upper administration is imperative to the successful implementation and operation of a quality management program. Physicians and employees must believe that the program is designed to improve patient care and is supported at the highest levels of the institution. If the program is seen as a passing fad, neither physicians nor employees will devote energy to it guaranteeing its failure. Investment must be made at the top level of the organization to ensure commitment at lower levels.

Once the commitment of senior management is secured, establishing practice policies and initiating changes in practice patterns must originate in the medical staff. The medical staff will not accept nor abide by practice policies that are imposed upon them by others; ownership of the program must reside with the medical staff. The responsibility of administration must be to provide direction, education, tools and personnel and delegate change authority to the medical staff.

Responsibility for undertaking patient satisfaction surveys and incorporating the survey results into hospital operations should reside with the quality management program. Patient satisfaction surveys address the entire scope of hospital operations. It is essential that every department understand their role in producing positive responses and buy-in to the goals, methodology and interpretation of the survey. The quality management program should provide the required training, disseminate and interpret results, work with departments to develop and implement solutions for any sources of dissatisfaction and monitor any changes after they are initiated.

Determining what to measure to evaluate the technical expectations is as complex as medicine practice itself. Many institutions will not have the expertise to initiate and monitor practice standards as described above and should begin by focusing on easily measured factors such as infection rates, medication errors, readmissions, LOS, etcetera. After developing expertise and gaining credibility, the quality management program should expand into practice policy development and examining deviations from these patterns. Practice policies should be developed according to the importance of the medical treatment to the patient and institution and aim to reduce deviations from the standard.

Patient satisfaction measures the patient perception of the care process and what they considered outstanding, acceptable or unacceptable service. Surveys should poll patients on the institution's hotel functions including access to services, convenience of parking, registration functions, room attributes and quality of meals, its medical functions including physician, nursing and ancillary services and an overall evaluation. Typical survey instruments use a 5-point Likert scale where patients assess the quality of each factor from 5 – highly satisfied to 1- highly dissatisfied. Comparing survey ratings against historical results and/or comparable institutions will determine institution performance and need for change.

Measuring the actual health delivery process and outcome requires more sophistication. Statistical process control is the application of statistical techniques to determine when a process is operating up to expectations (in-control) and when adjustments must be made to meet standards (out-of-control). All processes are subject to variation and will from one time period to another vary in the amount and quality of output produced. Statistics is essential to determining when a system is in-control or out-of-control and establishing credibility in the eyes of health care personnel that the program has been established on a solid methodological foundation.

In statistics the central limit theorem states as a sample size becomes large and each observation is independently selected from a population having a mean μ and standard deviation σ, the sampling distribution tends towards a normal distribution with a mean μ and standard deviation σ_x. The mean measures the value around which observations tend to cluster and their magnitude. The standard deviation measures the range or dispersion of the observations. Using the mean and standard deviation a normal distribution (bell curve) can be constructed. The bell curve allows us to predict how many observations should fall within various ranges of the mean, for example within one standard deviation 67 percent of all observations should fall, within two 95 percent. Conversely beyond two standards deviations there is only a 5 percent chance that a sample mean that falls outside this range comes from a normal or in-control process and the difference between the mean and the sample mean is due to pulling a non-representative sample.

Given a sample mean more than two standard deviations from the desired mean, we can be confident that the underlying process requires investigation and potentially corrective action. This tool can be used to evaluate health care processes over time, patients or providers. For example, we may want the length of stay for DRG 105 Cardiac Valve Procedures without Cardiac Catherization to be approximately equal to the Medicare geometric mean of 12.7 days. Figure 2.3 shows that our LOS is 13.0, is this something we need to investigate and implement corrective action or do the outliers of 10 and 16 days require action?

Figure 2.3 – DRG 105 – Length of Stay

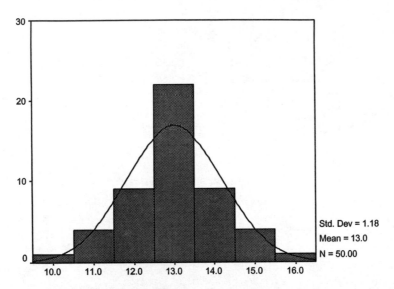

Std. Dev = 1.18
Mean = 13.0
N = 50.00

Answering this question requires us to determine if the deviation is statistically significant or if it is due to chance, that is the process is in-control but we drew a bad sample. The standard deviation of 1.18 means that 67 percent of all cases should be hospitalized between 11.82 and 14.18 days, likewise 95 percent of these admissions should last between 10.64 and 15.36 days. In this case it does not appear that our distribution of cases is abnormal so we will simply continue monitoring.

Lets assume another treatment plan for cardiac valve patients produces the histogram shown in figure 2.4. The means for both processes are the same, 13 days, but the standard deviations are different. As stated earlier, narrow dispersions are preferred to wide dispersions, given a choice between treatment A with a standard deviation of 1.18 and treatment B with a standard deviation of 1.62, treatment A is preferable given similar outcomes. Treatment A shows greater consistency in the underlying production process while B indicates there is a greater difference in how patients are cared for and how long they require care. We may want to investigate why different approaches are used if similar outcomes are achieved but very different utilization of resources are required to achieve these outcomes. In addition, we may want to investigate the cases discharged after 8 and 17 days to make sure that their length of stays were appropriate. The goal of quality health care requires that patients not be discharged too quickly or too late.

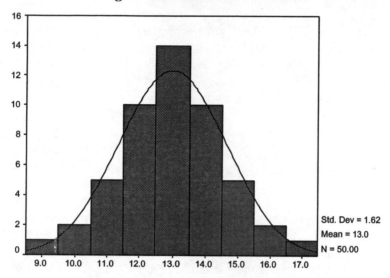

Figure 2.4 - DRG 105 - Process B

Std. Dev = 1.62
Mean = 13.0
N = 50.00

Correction efforts must be limited to those deviations that require system adjustments to produce the output we desired. This requires a system that can identify variations that are part of normal process operation and target only those deviations that are unlikely to be the result of chance. Statistics provides a defensible tool to identify quality problems, that is deviation in treatment patterns that suggest potential problems in a production process requiring remedial action.

Implementing a statistically based quality management process is a four-step process. The first step is data collection. Samples must be drawn to determine the sample mean, the measure of central tendency, and the sample standard deviation, the measure of dispersion.

The second step is to compare the sample mean and standard deviation against the desired outcome. No process produces the same output over time but during some periods will produce above expectations and in other periods below expectations. Statistical process control takes these deviations and breaks them into natural variation, that is expected changes based on random, naturally occurring changes in the production process and assignable variation, those changes above and beyond normal expectations which indicate a potential problem in the production process. Assignable variations indicate that there is some deficiency in labor, supplies, equipment and/or the process itself that is causing it to produce below expectations. This non-random variation requires us to pinpoint and correct the factor or factors that produce sub-optimal performance.

Control charts are used to identify when investigation and correction are needed. A control chart is built with tolerances, upper and lower limits in which a process can fluctuate before investigation is required. These limits are determined statistically, how many standard deviations should we allow the process to fluctuate within and still consider it to be operating normally or in-control. Tolerances are established with reference to the cost of failure, the higher the cost of failure the smaller the tolerance. If an out-of-control situation would produce dire health outcomes or exorbitant costs smaller tolerances are used so that investigation and correction are undertaken often to avoid these adverse results.

The x-bar chart examines central tendency (mean) to determine if the process is producing the expected outcomes on average i.e. is the average length of day increasing, decreasing or stable and does it fall within an acceptable range? The R chart examines that variability (range) of a production process, average length of stay may fall within the defined limits but is the process stable? Is length of stay increasing for one group of patients or one practitioner and decreasing for others? While the average is stable the diverging performance may require investigation and correction. Figure 2.5 presents the control charts for treatment plan B for DRG 105 patients.

Figure 2.5 – Control Charts, x-bar and R charts

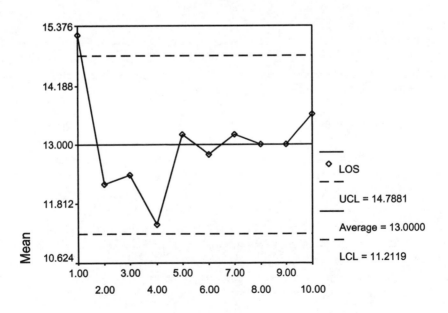

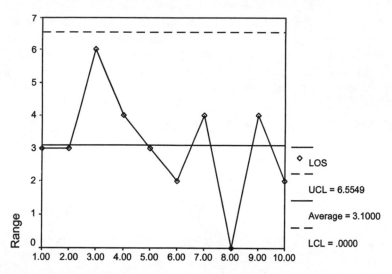

The x-bar chart shows the primary concern is the first sample of patients, this sample has a mean outside our tolerance range indicating that investigation into the cause of the high length of stay is needed. The other nine samples fall within defined limits and show no pattern. The cause of the variance in the first sample could be the health care personnel, equipment, a change in the treatment plan, the patients cared for or the time period when care was delivered. Further investigation is required, the control chart and identification of sample one simply provide a starting point for the investigation into the causes of the deviation. The R chart shows the variance in all samples fall within the established limits and there is no pattern to data points.

The third step is feedback. After an assignable variation is identified, the involved parties should be brought into the process to determine if corrective action is required. The parties should first be informed of the process used to identify the variation. Their expertise and cooperation are essential to determining if corrective action is needed and if so what should be done to prevent the deviation and how any necessary change should be implemented. Identification of assignable variation is not the end of the process but the beginning, identifying the reason for the variation is more difficult. Management science utilizes many tools to identify system problems including cause and effect diagrams, pareto charts and flow charts to pinpoint causes of sub-optimal performance.

Figure 2.6 shows a cause and effect diagram, this diagram identifies a problem and then lists potential causes for the problem along the major spines. In our example a high length of stay could be due to labor,

41

equipment, facilities or the treatment process. After major causes are identified, minor causes are then listed, for example, labor problems that contribute to a prolonged length of stay may arise from the medical staff, nurses, technicians or administrative personnel. The purpose of the diagram is to produce an exhaustive set of potential causes to sub-optimal performance so that the ultimate solution will encompass all contributing factors and not simply identify and attempt to rectify a single factor.

Figure 2.6 – Cause and Effect Diagram

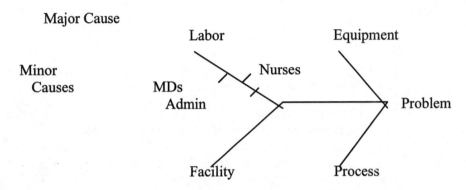

The fourth step is correction. After the reason(s) have been identified, training and controls should be implemented to prevent a reoccurrence of the problem. The main responsibility lies with the employees operating the process but quality management personnel must be vigilant in monitoring that corrective action is taken and maintain. For more detailed information on statistical process control the reader should examine Heizer and Render (1996).

Once an organization becomes comfortable with this process it should use its growing expertise to strive for continuous improvement in the quality of care delivered. Use of the Plan-Do-Check-Act (PDCA) cycle is one way of reaching this goal. This process is a trial and learning model designed to reduce variation and continuously improve quality. The four steps are documentation of the current process and outcomes to establish benchmarks (Plan), evaluation to determine where improvements can be made and implementation of changes (Do), re-evaluation of outcomes (Check) and implementation of other changes (Act). It is a revolving cycle of evaluation and change to determine what works and what doesn't. The PDCA cycle is designed to produce the best possible patient outcome through continual monitoring of processes and outcomes.

Finance

Quality isn't free. The question is: is high quality health care cheaper than low quality health care? Many note that current reimbursement systems pay on the basis of what is done and do not necessarily require things to done right. Besides quality insensitive reimbursement systems, hospitals have little incentive to pursue a high quality marketing strategies when patients are often unable to judge high and low quality care. In spite of these problems there are many reasons why standardization and high quality care should produce positive financial results for individual institutions and the U.S. health system.

Differences in practice style with no resulting change in health outcomes have been discussed. Phelps and Mooney (1992) suggest if average national utilization rates for the top 25 surgical procedures are correct and utilization of these services across the country could be reduced to the average the U.S. would have saved $6 billion in 1987 or roughly 1.2 percent of total health expenditure.

Uncertainty in medical practice produces over-utilization of care as physician engaged in defensive medicine, ordering more tests and procedures, to guard against malpractice claims. Zuckerman (1984) surveyed physicians and found that 41 percent claimed to perform more tests and 45 percent made more referrals to specialists due to malpractice concerns. Reynolds, Rizzo and Gonzalez (1987) estimate that defensive medical practices added between $12 and $14 billion dollars in physician services in 1984. The added practice cost plus the cost of malpractice insurance accounts for 16 percent to 18 percent of all physician expenditures. Quality management and practice standards could reduce these costs by establishing objective "best practice" standards that would increase practitioner confidence that they met their standard of care duties.

Beyond the societal cost savings presented by higher quality health care there is abundant evidence that individual institutions can institute programs that will reduce costs and improve their financial performance. Institutions are obviously sensitive to reducing the amount of services performed if that will lead to lower hospital revenues. Hospitals, however, have an incentive to pursue quality initiatives that reduce the cost of care by more efficient management of resources. Hospitals should strive to render the same number of patient care episodes but manage the delivery of care so that fewer resources are required to produce positive patient outcomes.

Todaro and Schott-Baer (2000) report that clinical pathways at two hospitals

43

produced reductions in length of stay and total episode costs. In addition to these reductions, the hospitals reduced clinical and surgical complications. Hughes (1998) reviewed multiple quality initiatives and found cost reducing opportunities across health care organizations. The hospitals reviewed targeted specific health conditions or processes for attention and achieved annual savings between $312,000 and $39,133,413. Given the reimbursement systems used by Medicare and managed care organizations it is clear that the majority of these cost reductions enhanced the operating results of these organizations.

Although many health care personnel are apprehensive about cost control, these initiatives expand the ability of organizations to provide patient care. If quality management reduces costs, it frees resources to be used for other services. No one gains if health care resources are used in a manner that does not improve patient outcomes or where the cost of the service is greater than the benefit created. Board members are responsible for insuring that their organization's resources are applied to those areas where they are both effectively and efficiently used.

Conclusion

This chapter introduced hospital board members to quality management programs and the role that practice policies will play in determining how medical care is delivered. Much of the concern over practice policies has to do with how they impact the autonomy and decision-making processes of physicians. There are wide differences in the goals and consequences of standards, guidelines and options and when each should be used. Usage will be determined by our understanding of the effectiveness of medical treatments and the wishes of patients. In the majority of cases our understanding of these two issues will favor the use of guidelines and options insuring that physicians will continue to exercise broad professional judgment.

Beyond the immediate goal of improving patient care the long-range goal of quality management programs is to increase our understanding of patient preferences and clinical effectiveness. The chapter introduces both statistical process control and the PDCA cycle as means of monitoring clinical effectiveness and improving patient outcomes. Physicians trained in the scientific method, that is taught to evaluate evidence before making decisions, need to see quality management programs as based on a scientifically and statistically firm foundation and designed to assist them in patient care. These programs must produce information that allows physicians to evaluate and change their practice styles to achieve better patient outcomes.

Quality management thus will not only facilitate the institution goal of providing the best possible patient care but in addition these programs offer the benefits of building teamwork among hospital employees who are all focused on improving patient care and the potential for improving the institution's operating results. The board member's responsibility is to see that his or her institution focuses not only on doing the right things but concentrates on doing things right.

NOTES:

Chapter 3

Maximizing Employee Productivity

By: Marc C. Marchese, Ph.D.
Associate Professor of Human Resources Management
King's College

Maximizing Employee Productivity

The basic definition of an organization is a collection of people working collectively toward a common goal. To achieve the goal, the company needs its people to be highly productive. The productivity of its people will be greatly affected by how those people are managed. The key to effective management is creating a high performance work environment in the organization. This chapter will focus on the critical parts of such an environment.

To create a high performance work environment three major factors must be considered thoroughly. These three factors are the environment, the company's human resources philosophy and key human resources practices in the organization. All three of these factors are equally important in affecting employee productivity.

The environment in which a company exists is crucial to understanding the keys to managing its employees. There are so many aspects of the environment that impact how an organization should treat its employees that to ignore the environment is a recipe for disaster. In this section the top five factors of the environment affecting employee productivity will be discussed.

ENVIRONMENT

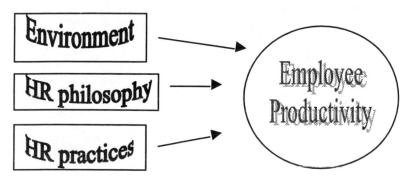

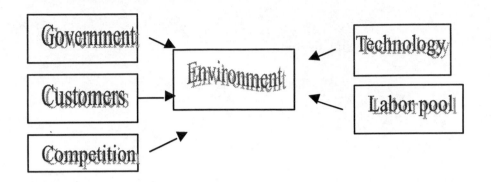

[1] Governmental Influences

In today's litigious society no discussion of how a company treats its employees, former employees, and applicants would be complete without mentioning the numerous legal influences. There are many state and federal regulations affecting virtually all aspects of the employment process. Moreover, multinational organizations have to account for various legal systems across national borders.

To give you an idea of the countless ways government regulations may impact an organization, a brief sample of some legal employment issues follows. To start, in the process of defining job requirements the Americans with Disabilities Act requires identifying "essential job functions" to help assess whether a person with a disability may be qualified for employment. In advertising open positions the manner in which the help wanted ad is written (e.g., using masculine pronouns) could provide evidence of sex discrimination under the Civil Rights Act. Further, in the hiring process, using unproven requirements (e.g., high school diploma) to weed out applicants can be seen by the courts as racially biased. Additionally, once on the job employee compensation can be affected by the Fair Labor Standards Act (e.g., overtime pay, exempt v. nonexempt classification). Also, promotional decisions influenced by subjective criteria (e.g., ability to learn) might be perceived as a form of age discrimination under the Age Discrimination in Employment Act. In addition, terminating employees can be scrutinized for discriminatory intent. For example, letting go of an employee for excessive absences due to pregnancy may violate the Pregnancy Discrimination Act or the Family Medical Leave Act. Furthermore, numerous government regulatory agencies (e.g., EEOC, OSHA, NLRB) have various policies and procedures as well as legal authority (e.g., OSHA authority to conduct safety inspections) that must be accounted for by companies. Overall, legal entanglements can destroy any productive culture.

[2] Consumers

In any highly competitive marketplace successful organizations are the companies that know how to satisfy their customers. Attracting, motivating and retaining employees that know how to meet and exceed client expectations is therefore vital. To identify the characteristics of the ideal employee, organizations have to first make sure they have a strong understanding of their customers. Consumers for a given organization can be quite diverse regardless if the marketplace is local, national or global.

In examining the customers for a given organization, several aspects should be considered. To begin with, the language differences among one's customers will have an impact on identifying productive employees. If an organization knows that a considerable portion of its customers do not speak English, then the company is faced with either trying to recruit bilingual employees or spend training dollars on foreign language skills. Further, if the company has locations outside the United States it will have to decide whether it would be better to recruit from the immediate area, capitalizing on the familiarity of the applicants with the local culture, or to use expatriates who may have stronger familiarity with the organization and its goals.

In addition to language differences among a company's clients, demographic and cultural characteristics should be assessed as well. The age, race, sex, and socioeconomic makeup of the client base could influence targeting ideal employees. Diversity in the customer base may be best serviced by a diverse workforce or at least a workforce that is skilled at handling a wide range of customers.

A third aspect of the customer base that should be examined is their values or preferences regarding the organization's market. Highly productive employees will know what the customers really want (whether it be wide selection, low prices, high quality, etc.). In addition, if the given company is in a market in which consumer tastes change on a regular basis, ideal employees will need to be flexible to these changes as will the company. In conclusion, a company that understands its customers will understand and develop highly productive employees.

[3] Competition

Competition affects organizations in countless ways, including several ways that can affect employee productivity. To begin with, an organization's competitors will influence the company's ability to attract the best applicants. As the nation's unemployment remains low, the struggle to obtain highly qualified employees while at the same time attempting to contain labor costs is a challenge. Starting salaries as well as the benefits package (especially in the areas of health care coverage and retirement packages) across organizations in a given industry will be compared and negotiated by the most desirable applicants.

In addition to attracting qualified applicants, competitors will also influence an organization's ability to retain highly productive employees. Private employment agencies, executive recruiters and "headhunters" are often used to persuade the best employees of one company to move to a competitor for the promise of better compensation, greater responsibilities (e.g., a vice-president position) or more desirable quality of life issues (e.g., telecommuting).

A third manner in which competitors can affect an organization's employee productivity is through a process known as benchmarking. Benchmarking is a system by which a company compares its performance on certain critical business operations to others in the same market who are considered the "best" at that given operation. Typically benchmarking is a quantitative approach to see how one organization stacks up to its competition. In terms of employee productivity, benchmarking has been used to assess business operations such as turnover rates, product quality, units produced per employee, and even employee theft rates. Once an organization evaluates how far apart it is from other organizations, then changes (e.g., performance improvement goals, implementation plans) may be made to achieve the standards the organization wishes to reach.

[4] Emerging Technology

In this information age technology is constantly changing. Telecommunications, medical research instrumentation, artificial intelligence initiatives and robotics are just a few of the areas in which technology has rapidly advanced. The breadth and depth of technological change is quite impressive. All organizations are affected by technological change regardless of whether the industry is service or manufacturing.

Technological change can influence a productive workforce in a handful of ways. To start with, technological skills should be a strong factor in the recruiting needs of an organization. Finding applicants with the proper education and experience to operate technology is a given. Moreover, as technology changes, job requirements will also change. Companies are faced with deciding when resources should be devoted to training existing employees on the new technology and/or when resources should be devoted

50

to finding new employees skilled in the latest technology. Further, technological advances may eliminate certain jobs in an organization or at least reduce the number of positions needed for a given job (e.g., number of bank tellers needed after the advent of ATMs). If positions or jobs are eliminated, then the company has to decide if those affected employees will be released, which in turn can negatively affect the morale and productivity of the other employees who remain in their jobs, or if they will be reassigned, which in turn may necessitate higher training expenditures to prepare the employees for the new assignments. Finally, technological advancements can also create new jobs in an organization (e.g., web masters). A cost-benefit analysis will be needed to evaluate the value of adding more jobs in the company.

[5] Labor Pool

The final aspect of the environment that has a significant impact on employee productivity is the labor pool. This segment of the environment has the most direct influence on employee performance compared to the other four factors simply because this is the source of new employees for an organization.

The increasing diversity of the labor force is well known. Diversity as a concept can be interpreted quite broadly. When referring to the labor force diversity is often mentioned in terms of greater racial and ethnic diversity. The diversity of the labor pool also includes an aging workforce, a greater participation rate of women (including working mothers), as well as more foreign-born workers. Moreover, two diverging trends are also occurring in the labor pool. The percentage of employees with college degrees is increasing as well as the percentage of illiterate employees.

The diversity issues mentioned above present several challenges to businesses that can definitely influence employee productivity. To maximize employee productivity it is important that the employees are a cohesive team. Knowledge needs to be shared. Thus, cooperation must be the norm. Attaining a cohesive work unit is more difficult when employees perceive other employees as different, strange or threatening. To overcome some of the difficulties of a diverse workforce, effective organizations need to devote time and money towards building positive work relationships. These initiatives may include such things as: cultural awareness training, informal opportunities for socialization, harassment education (whether it be based on sex, race and/or age), conflict management, and language skills education.

51

In addition to the labor force changes mentioned above, another substantial change in the workforce is a change in work values. The priorities of today's worker have been altered. Issues such as balancing work and family demands, flexible scheduling (e.g., flextime), greater time off, task variety and opportunities to develop are becoming more prominent in the labor force. Organizations that can satisfy these desires will have an easier time attracting, retaining and motivating their employees.

In conclusion, the environment in which an organization operates can significantly impact the productivity of that given organization. Companies that do a thorough job analyzing and interpreting the implications of the environment are much more likely to maximize employee productivity.

Human Resources Philosophy

The second major factor that has a considerable impact on maximizing employee productivity is the organization's view of its employees. An effective human resource philosophy is one in which employees are considered a valuable resource that if managed properly can be a strategic advantage for the company. HR philosophies can differ across organizations: however, four basic elements comprise most human resource philosophies: effective communication throughout the organization, meaningful rewards for the most productive employees, opportunities for employee development, and a culture of respect.

[1] Effective Communication

In today's workplace it is rare to find any job that is isolated from other jobs in the organization. Even if a job is performed in an isolated location, most likely the functions associated with that job are affected by and/or affect other jobs in the company. Interdependence of jobs within organizations is commonplace. To maximize employee productivity in an interdependent work environment effective communication is required. Employees need to know what certain other employees are doing and why they are doing it, which in turn will affect how that given employee will perform his or her job to enhance work performance.

Moreover, more and more organizations are moving towards team-based initiatives. If employees are expected to operate within a team framework they need to communicate with each other quite often. As the old adage goes, "there's no 'I' in team." Without effective communication in a team, there will be limited cooperation, regular conflict, missed opportunities and duplication of efforts. Team productivity will be greatly constrained without effective communication.

The diversity of the labor pool was discussed in the previous section of this chapter. Diversity in progressive organizations is considered an advantage rather than a potential stumbling block. A diverse workforce has people of various backgrounds with a wide variety of skills, interests and experiences. This concept is illustrated in the case of a small manufacturing company that was losing customers because they were unable to recruit bilingual customer service representatives. After several weeks passed they happened to discover a long-term manufacturing employee was bilingual and was willing to switch jobs. Shortly thereafter the company discovered several manufacturing employees who had similar skills and interests. If the company had communicated better with its employees, it would never have lost customers for this reason. By practicing effective communication, companies can capitalize of the diversity of their workforces to make more informed decisions, generate new ideas and ultimately improve organizational performance.

[2] Meaningful Reward System

Another critical aspect of a company's view of its workforce is the manner by which it rewards its employees. Employees quickly learn what the organization really cares about by the ways in which the company decides such issues as pay increases, advancement decisions, training and development opportunities, allocating authority on special projects, and other forms of rewards.

In an organization that is attempting to maximize employee productivity, the reward system must be aligned with the organization's goals and objectives. If the company's primary objectives are such things as improving customer service, enhancing product quality, greater on-time delivery, or increasing customers, then the reward system should incorporate these goals in a central way. Too often businesses have objectives such as these, however rewards are based primarily on longevity, attendance, subjective ratings of personality traits or strategic friendships. In these cases employee motivation rapidly moves away from focusing on performance to other less crucial facets of work.

In addition to creating a reward system clearly connected to organizational decisions, there are other aspects that affect the value of a reward system. If the company truly sees its employees as a valuable resource, then the reward system needs to show employees that the organization is serious in rewarding desired performance. Employees that meet and exceed performance standards must know their reward is significant (e.g., clear pay raise that is evident even if it is spread out over 26 pay periods) and significantly greater than those employees who failed to meet performance standards. If the top performers in a certain job category receive pay increases only a percentage or two higher than the across the board pay raise, then the motivating properties of the pay raises are greatly diminished. Why would an employee bother to push his or her productivity when the difference is minimal compared to other employees doing marginal work?

A final aspect of a meaningful reward system connects to the first aspect of an effective HR philosophy. For any reward system to function properly employees have to know what the system is, understand how the system is implemented and believe that the system is fair. Communication is essential for these three tasks to be accomplished. Employees need to have the system spelled out in writing some way (e.g., memo, Intranet link). In addition, group or individual meetings for employees to review the system must take place. Finally, employees need to have some way to voice their ideas, concerns and/or questions about the system for the system to be fully understood and accepted by the company's workforce. A company's commitment to a meaningful reward system can have a considerable influence on maximizing employee productivity.

[3] Employee Development

This component of a strong HR philosophy can be considered a subset of the previous component. Companies that provide numerous opportunities for employees to grow are in a very meaningful way rewarding their employees. As indicated in the section describing the labor pool, employees in the 21st century value opportunities to develop.

When considering employee development initiatives organizations should distinguish between employee development alternatives intended to maximize employee productivity (short and long-term in nature) and employee development alternatives that function as a perk for employees. For example, many companies allow employees to obtain a college degree at the company's expense. If employees can pursue any major they wish, then this type of development program is clearly a perk. Employees may pursue degrees unrelated to their job (e.g., an accounts payable clerk receiving a B.S. in elementary education), and once they graduate may leave the organization to fulfill their vocational interests. This type of program is generous and may boost retention (at least in the short-term) as well as morale, however it is likely to have little impact on improving employee productivity. It may actually hurt productivity, because the employee is devoting more time to their education than to going above and beyond on the job.

Employee development programs intended to increase employee productivity need to take into account several factors. To begin with, employee development programs, like reward systems, should be aligned with organizational objectives. Companies need to address questions such as: What kind of workforce do we want? Do we want our employees to be experts in a specialized component of our production or service process? Or do we want employees that are flexible, multi-skilled and innovative? The answer to questions like these will have obvious implications to the types of development programs a company should offer as well as which employees will have access to which programs.

Meaningful reward systems including effective employee development programs can be quite costly for organizations, and deciding how much time and money is needed to implement these programs successfully is not easy. In these turbulent times of global competition, emerging technology and changing customer preferences, it is critical that a company has a workforce that is motivated, eager to learn and committed to accomplishing organizational objectives.

[4] Respect

The final component of a HR philosophy that is related to enhancing employee productivity is developing and maintaining a culture of respect in the workplace. Respect is a very broad concept that can include the other three components in the section. Companies that believe in open communication, meaningful rewards for employees and providing opportunities for employees to grow and develop create a workplace that respects its employees. Respect in the workplace includes other aspects as well. Employees who feel respected by their employer, their supervisors and their coworkers are much more likely to care about their job and therefore more likely to work hard.

Organizations that want employees to know that they are respected should focus on three main areas: fairness, trust and power. Perceived fairness in the workplace can be affected by virtually any program or policy. Additionally, perceived fairness has two main components: process and outcome. Process refers to the manner in which the policy or program is carried out. Is the program implemented fairly? For example, in matters dealing with employee discipline, is there a consistent manner in which employee problems are investigated or do friendships affect how seriously complaints are processed? Another example could be in the area of performance reviews. Are performance evaluations based on objective job-relevant criteria or based on subjective supervisor ratings of personality? Outcome refers to the end result of the program or policy. Even if the process is fair, the outcome could be viewed as unjust. As indicated earlier, a reward system that is implemented well (fair process) but yields small differences in pay between marginal and top performers would be perceived as unfair. An employee discipline program that consistently investigates employee problems could be perceived as unfair if the penalties are severe for minor infractions of company rules (e.g., two incidents of lateness over a 12 month period resulting in termination). An unfair workplace can be evidence of a company that does not respect its employees.

Trust is the second component of respect. Open and honest communication in the workplace demonstrates to employees that the company trusts them enough to share vital information. Employee development programs also show employees that the company trusts them. Opportunities to grow and develop communicates to employees that the organization trusts that they will take the programs seriously and apply it to the workplace. There is a clear message that these initiatives benefit both the employee and the organization. The company is making a commitment to the employee, which enhances the trust the employee has for the organization.

Power is the third aspect of respect. If an organization respects its employees, then it should be willing to empower its workforce. Giving employees the responsibility to make decisions regarding their jobs demonstrates that the company respects the employees' talents. Supervisors are viewed as facilitators rather than dictators. Employees will be developing their decision-making skills in addition to their technical expertise.

In conclusion, fairness, open and honest communication, and trusting employees through empowerment are ways to show employees respect in the workplace, which should ultimately lead to a productive workplace. Add in a meaningful reward system and opportunities for employee development and the company will have an effective HR philosophy that will promote a high performance work environment.

Human Resources Practices

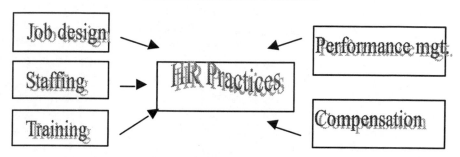

After an organization has examined the environment for opportunities and threats from the government, customers, competition, emerging technology and the labor pool as well as developed a human resources philosophy that values effective communication, meaningful rewards, development opportunities and respect in the workplace, the last part of maximizing employee productivity is to align key HR practices. There are numerous functions and issues that fall under the realm of human resources, however five major areas are the most critical to affecting employee performance. These five HR areas are job design, staffing, training, performance management and compensation.

[1] Job Design

The foundation of human resources management is job design. To achieve organizational goals, work must be divided into manageable pieces. Typically, work is divided into divisions, departments, and ultimately jobs. Defining jobs is central to maximizing employee productivity in the following ways:

(a) Establishing the relevance of the job requirements in relation to meeting organizational objectives.
(b) Establishing the qualifications of job candidates in the staffing process.

(c) Preventing duplication of activities across jobs.

(d) Identifying links with other jobs, which can then be used to enhance communication and coordination in the workplace.

(e) Assisting in creating performance standards for a given job.

(f) Creating training objectives for new hires for a given job.

(g) Establishing the value of jobs in the organizational hierarchy, which in turn can affect the compensation system in the company.

Based upon the above-mentioned reasons, the importance of job design is evident. There are numerous methods of conducting a thorough job analysis with numerous advantages and disadvantages of each approach. It is beyond the scope of this chapter to discuss the specifics of the various methods of job analysis, however there are a few other issues worth mentioning.

In defining the duties, responsibilities and tasks associated with a given job, the organization may also want to reconsider the efficiency of the workplace. Are there ways in which the work environment can be redesigned to reduce wasted efforts? If there are certain jobs that are quite interdependent, can the work sites of these jobs be moved physically closer to each other? If the employee in a given job regularly uses certain supplies or materials, can these materials be moved next to the person's workstation? In completing a task, are there particular activities that do not add value to the process and thus can be eliminated?

In addition, the field of ergonomics looks at redesigning a job to make completing tasks less physically stressful on the employee. This can reduce workplace injuries and ultimately improve employee productivity. Finally, job enrichment initiatives can be considered for a given job to improve job satisfaction and performance. For example, increasing responsibilities for a particular job can be viewed by the employee as more challenging and thus more rewarding, which in turn can translate into higher job performance.

[2] Staffing

Once the job requirements are clearly defined, the next challenge for a company is finding the right person for the job. The staffing process has a considerable amount of complexity. Human resources planning should play a key role in the staffing process. Organizations need to forecast how many employees will be needed in the near future (next 6 months) as well as down the road (two to five years). Numerous factors will influence these projections: turnover rates, consumer demand, economic indicators (e.g., low interest rates), retirement benefits, and strategic organizational decisions (e.g., expansion plans, eliminating a product line, merger). When this process is complete, the organization will have a good idea of how many employees will be needed in various jobs across the company within a certain time frame.

Next, the company has to decide to what extent it wants to be committed to the people that fill these job openings. Independent contractors, full-time temporary help, part-time employees and even outsourcing particular functions may be more effective options to meet the company's needs than hiring traditional full-time employees. The following questions need to be answered: Are these staffing needs long or short-term in nature? Are these jobs critical to attracting and retaining customers? What will be the impact of hiring contingent workers on our full-time staff? Employee productivity can be diminished if employees perceive that the organization is more concerned about cutting costs than about developing and rewarding quality workers.

If the company decides the best way to fill the company's staffing needs is through hiring traditional full-time employees, the next step is to develop a high quality applicant pool. Organizations need to first decide whether current employees should be given the opportunity to apply for job openings before external candidates will be considered. Internal recruiting is related to several aspects of an effective HR philosophy. It shows that the company wants to develop its employees. Further, it shows respect for the employees. It communicates to employees that the company is committed to them.

If the company decides to recruit externally there are numerous recruiting options ranging from the traditional help wanted ad in the local paper to posting openings in a virtual community on the Internet. The relevant labor market (e.g. local, national, international) needs to be identified before recruiting methods are selected. Further, the recruiting process should clearly communicate desired qualifications to avoid receiving countless job inquiries from unqualified applicants. Finally, current employees should be solicited for recruiting ideas since they are working in the given field and may have knowledge of valuable recruiting sources.

At this point, the company has to select the best applicants based upon the number of job openings. Again the company has many options ranging from traditional selection methods (e.g., evaluating application forms and conducting background checks) to relatively new selection procedures (e.g., behaviorally-based interviewing, computer-mediated testing). As with recruiting, the selection process should attempt to include current employees. Employees have the experience to truly understand the job requirements. In addition, employees will have to work with the new hires. If employees are involved in the process, they will be more comfortable with the chosen applicants and will feel more responsible for their success. Practically speaking this should help with socializing and educating the new hires in the workplace. It is highly inefficient for a company to spend time and money on recruitment and selection if the new hires leave after a short time because they are not accepted on the job.

The key factor in developing the selection process is job relevance. In what way does the information obtained in this selection method (e.g., interviewing) relate to successful job performance? Is there an established relationship between how well applicants perform on this selection component (e.g., years of previous work experience on resumé) and how well they perform on the job? This process of scrutinizing the job relevance of selection components will eliminate wasted time and money, produce a valid selection system which can used if necessary to defend the company in case of a lawsuit (recall governmental influences in the environment), yield highly qualified employees, and ultimately enhance productivity in the workplace.

[3] Training

After the selection process is complete, the next HR function influencing employee performance is training. There are many types of training, all of which have clear connections to employee motivation, retention and productivity. Shortly after the employee is hired there needs to be some type of orientation. New hires need to be made aware of the organization's goals, history, physical layout, key policies, overview of goods/services, and key leaders. In addition, some organizations, to help with retention as well as career development, implement a mentoring program for employees. Mentoring can be an excellent way for employees to be made aware of development opportunities, to learn about the informal workings of the organization, to develop a support network inside the company, and to learn about strategies to help employees balance work and family issues.

In addition to orientation, every company should engage in some form of operational training. Operational training refers to teaching employees about specific aspects of their job. Even if the new hire is highly qualified, there are usually several company-specific aspects to any job that the new hire must learn to be productive. This type of training is often done on-the-job through employee shadowing or coaching.

60

Another type of training is informational training. In this type of training employees learn about new developments in the workplace. This training can include things such as educating employees about new policies (e.g., new grievance system) or about new services the company is planning to offer to customers in the near future. There are many options in communicating new information to employees (e.g., large-scale meetings, videoconferencing, Intranet link).

The most important type of training related to maximizing employee productivity is high leverage training. In this type of training, training objectives are directly linked to organizational objectives. For example, if the organization is embracing total quality management (TQM), then training employees on TQM is essential to meeting this goal. As discussed in the competition section of the environment, benchmarking is often used in this type of strategic training to establish training expectations.

In sum, no matter how qualified an employer's workforce is to do its job, employees need help fitting into the organization through effective orientation and mentoring programs. They also need to learn company specific processes to do their job, to be made aware of changes in the organization, and to be trained in accordance with strategic organizational objectives to maximize employee productivity.

[4] Performance Management and [5] Compensation

Although these two HR functions are often discussed separately, if a company is serious about maximizing employee productivity these two areas should be intertwined. Further, these two HR functions are closely connected to developing a "meaningful reward system." Many of the issues that were presented in that section of this chapter are relevant here as well.

A company that wants to maximize employee productivity first needs to establish productivity expectations. These standards can be based on the job analysis findings, benchmarking research, and employee input. Once the standards are established, an objective system to measure performance needs to be created. This is not easy since it is often difficult to quantify the most important aspects of many jobs. Employee input and multiple sources of information (e.g., peer ratings, self ratings, supervisor ratings) may be needed to make a fair performance evaluation system.

After the evaluation system is in place, the employee should be afforded training opportunities to address performance problems. In addition, constructive feedback, given on a regular basis, should be communicated to

61

employees to keep them on track towards accomplishing performance standards. After a certain period of time (e.g., yearly, semi-annually) or after completion of a major task, employee productivity needs to be formally evaluated based upon the established system. In the formal evaluation, employees should be made aware of their level of performance on the various components. Strengths and weaknesses should be identified. Moreover, the employees should be allowed to voice their opinions of the factors that helped and hindered effective performance. This feedback from employees cannot only identify some obstacles to effective performance; it will also show that the organization values employees' ideas. The company wants to see the employees perform well and is interested in their input.

The compensation system should then be linked to this performance evaluation process. As discussed earlier, the most productive employees should be rewarded the most. Also, the rewards must be substantial. Keep in mind not all rewards need to be monetary. For many employees rewards such as recognition, greater discretion in completing work assignments, and flexibility (e.g., allowing a top performer to telecommute) are very meaningful. In addition, there should be significant differences between the top performers and the marginal performers. Further, the incentive compensation should occur shortly after the performance review. Employees need to see the connection between performance and rewards. Finally, organizations need to make all employees aware of the benefits of high performance. The magnitude and types of rewards for high productivity should be communicated in the workplace. Open and honest communication, as stated previously, is both respectful and well as potentially motivating to employees.

Overall, these five HR functions are critical to maximizing employee productivity. Companies first have to define job requirements and design jobs effectively to establish performance standards. Next, locating and identifying the best applicants is critical to creating a motivated competent workforce. Training and developing those employees is necessary to accomplish organizational objectives. Finally, evaluating and rewarding desired performance motivates employees to achieve top productivity levels.

Conclusion

The purpose of this chapter was to explore the numerous facets that affect employee productivity. The underlying assumption is that employees need to be perceived as a valuable resource. If employees are managed with this in mind, then the employer's workforce can reach maximum levels of productivity. The three main areas that affect employee performance are the environmental influences on the organization (government regulations, competition, customers, emerging technology, and the labor pool), the organization's philosophy toward its employees (open and honest communication, an effective reward system, opportunities for employee development, and a culture of respect) and certain human resource functions that directly relate to employee behavior (job analysis & design, staffing, training, performance management, and compensation).   In closing, maximizing employee productivity may be complex but the potential return on this investment is limitless.

NOTES:

64

Chapter 4

Ethics in Health Care Delivery
Ethics for Directors

By: Dan F. Kopen, M.D.

The information and knowledge contained throughout this book are essential to your ability to serve effectively as a director or trustee of a hospital, insurance carrier, foundation, academic health center, health service organization, or other related institution. However, the concepts discussed in this chapter lend the possibility of sustainable viability to the body of knowledge and expertise represented by the other sections. Without the principled application of the concepts subsumed under the rubric of ethics there is little or no likelihood of sustained success in furtherance of the mission of the organization that you have agreed to serve. The board, through its selection and oversight of the CEO as well as through its own deliberations and actions, sets the ethical tone of the organization.

The ends to which your institution has dedicated itself through its mission statement are no doubt worthy and respected intentions. Ethical considerations for the most part do not deal with the ends, which we will assume are honorable. Rather, ethics speaks directly to the means chosen to pursue those ends. There is no other arena of human endeavor wherein the ethical pursuit of objectives is more central or more crucial to the ultimate outcome than in health care. Failure to understand and apply ethical standards in the furtherance of institutional mission is arguably the single most frequent cause of shortcomings and failure among health care organizations. Furthermore, ethical considerations are not confined to human interactions. Ethics also weigh heavily and directly upon the ability to gather and analyze data, a critical first step in the process of understanding and improving performance.

This chapter will focus upon three key virtues and several related concepts with which most people should be familiar and with which people in positions of fiduciary responsibility need to be fully conversant. We will examine **truth, trust,** and **integrity.** Taken together these can be viewed as the three cardinal virtues of health care directorship. Comprehensive attention is paid to concepts involving truth because of the centrality of truth and the search for truth in all human undertakings. In particular, this discussion aims to improve your ability to seek truth and to avoid the pitfalls of manipulated meanings as people pursue personal and hidden agendas under the guise of searching for or having attained truth. This examination is followed by a review of the concept of the **learning ladder**, a schematic representation of the process of human learning that applies both to individuals and to institutions. Successful organizational learning depends upon the board's understanding of and commitment to truth, trust, and integrity. Finally, a short and accessible test in the form of an **ethical checklist** is offered to help you identify the presence or absence of ethical behaviors in your and your board's decision-making processes.

Truth

Truth is defined in the dictionary as "the body of real things, events, and facts." On the surface this is a deceptively simple concept most of us embrace without question. However, truth can be one of the most complex and elusive concepts we encounter. The vast expanse between the notion of the simple truth and the complexities embodied in knowing the whole truth serves as fertile ground for the emergence of both inadvertent and deliberate misunderstandings. These misunderstandings at an individual level can become multiplied many times over in organizational performance as each individual brings to the table a personal and therefore different perspective of "the truth" to bear on work processes. The result of disparate beliefs in the truth, often held subconsciously but also at times intentionally, is a major impediment to effective ethical process performance.

To embrace truth as a core value is to commit oneself to the full recognition and accurate communication of reality. Reality recognition, i.e. the truth, serves as the platform upon which we commence our undertakings, both private and public. Levels of achievement and ultimate success or failure are in large measure dependent upon our individual and collective abilities to seek and fully communicate truth. In the hierarchy of learning, the search for truth is the engine that powers the learning process. As Albert Einstein observed, "If we want to avoid defeat we must wish to know the truth and be courageous enough to act upon it."

A major problem confronting many of today's health care institutions is the wide gap between the truth of the enterprise and the perceptions of trustees and directors. This gap is often the result of deceptions by persons reporting to the board. At other times it is a result of the board's choosing to ignore the truth. This disparity can lead to forfeiture of fiduciary responsibility by the board. Absent the virtues of integrity and trustworthiness an individual's ability to pursue truth is severely impeded, while an organization is essentially precluded from truth recognition. The ability to constantly seek and report the truth is a hallmark of virtue in a leader. Truth is an ally of leadership founded on the principle of integrity. Truth is the enemy of

66

corrupt leadership. The fortunes of health care organizations often hinge on the ability and willingness of leadership to embrace truth as a cardinal principle.

In the search for truth we find the common ground of knowledge and information which, when shared and appropriately acted upon, allows an organization to continuously improve the quality of its goods and services. This in turn enhances the value of those goods and services, increases employee satisfaction, and bestows upon leadership a heightened sense of authenticity and legitimacy.

In order to better understand this topic, one needs to have some familiarity with the major theories of truth. Additionally, there exist an almost endless number of "truth tricks" that we play on ourselves and on each other, individually and collectively, both inadvertently and deliberately. It is essential for leaders and followers to understand and overcome these deceptions. The inability to identify and to report truth is probably the most common serious operational problem confronting organizations. This constitutes **truth decay**, the process of adulteration of the full, accurate, and timely communication of reality.

There are no fewer than nine different theories of truth referenced in *The Oxford Companion to Philosophy*. The four most commonly identified categories of truth as identified by Frederick F. Schmitt in *TRUTH: A Primer* should be part of the understanding of persons who assume the fiduciary responsibilities of a health care organization.

1. **Correspondence theory**: This is the most widely recognized and accepted formal expression of truth theory. According to the correspondence theory of truth, in order for a statement to be true it must correspond to fact or reality. Many feel that this is the most commonsense theory of truth. Truth depends upon how things are in relation to a statement, how closely the words correspond to reality. Beliefs are true in so far as they correspond to reality, and true statements are the links between reality and beliefs. The names most recognized and associated with this theory of truth are Aristotle and Bertrand Russell.

2. **Coherence theory**: This theory was originally proposed as an alternative to the correspondence theory. Coherence theory was developed by the rationalist metaphysicists and defines truth in terms of epistemic justification of knowledge. That is, a statement is true if it is coherent with other true statements as part of a comprehensive

67

system of true statements logically connected. The school of logical positivism adopted this theory of truth through the application of mathematics as a model. Religious truths are also largely determined by this model. The names Leibniz, Hegel and Bradley are associated with this theory.

3. **Pragmatic theory**: An invention of 19th century American philosophy and developed by Peirce, James and Dewey, this theory conceives of truth as a variable associated with a belief when confirmed by its usefulness to the holder of the belief. Truth is defined in terms of utility of belief to the believer, both behaviorally and cognitively. Central to this theory is the idea that truth matters. Problematic with this theory is the degree of relativism afforded by dependence upon the perception of utility held by the believer. This theory suffers more than the prior theories from the slippery slope phenomenon of progressive redefinition of truth in terms self-serving to the holder of a belief or hidden agenda.

4. **Deflationary theories**: Standing in stark contrast to the three substantive theories of truth outlined above are the deflationary theories. While the substantive theories assume that truth is real and an important ascriptive property of statements, the deflationary theories trivialize the concept of truth. Truth becomes a linguistic function captured by its relation to a truth-ascriber. Such theories include performative, redundancy, and prosentential theories. These hold that truth is at best only a technically useful concept and may even be dispensable. Deflationary theories of truth were developed in the 20th century and have developed a following among those espousing extreme forms of cultural relativism.

Something considered as true by one of the substantive theories will most often be held to be true by the other substantive theories. However, there are instances in which the theories will not reach agreement on the ascription of truth-value to an object, relationship, or belief. This brief sampler of truth theories is provided as an informational backdrop against which you can better understand the concept of truth and be wary of attempts to deflect attention from insistence on the search for truth by deflationists. The search for truth is central to creating a better future through generative leadership. Despite the attempts of deflationists to trivialize the concept, truth and the search for truth are essential and eternal aspects of human behavior.

Truth as Foundation

One of the most important aspects in which truth impacts individual and organizational performance is through its ability to reveal reality to those in policy-making and stewardship positions. The more accurate one's grasp of both historical and current reality, the fuller an understanding one can bring to bear on performance. The gap that exists between current conditions and future goals is of primary importance in organizational improvement. As described by Peter M. Senge in *The Fifth Discipline*, that perceived gap generates the creative tension which drives work processes. The more accurate the gap perception, i.e. the more truthful the recognition of current reality and the more realistic the future goals, the better positioned the organization is with respect to engaging appropriate resources in serving the mission of the organization. This holds for individuals as well as for groups. The truer one's beliefs, the more honest and accurate is the foundation upon which generative efforts are employed to narrow the disparity between what one has and what one would like to achieve. The more accurate the board's beliefs, the more appropriate will be the allocation of resources and greater overall achievement will accrue to the organization.

The human brain is not flawless and we concede that reality can neither be perfectly experienced nor perfectly understood. The one-to-two-hundred billion neurons and multi-trillion synapses (nerve to nerve connections) in the human brain are incapable of perfect knowledge. The price we pay for imperfect knowledge and imperfect communication is that we are forced to act on incomplete and often inaccurate information. The human species has evolved neurological mechanisms to selectively perceive and store data and to selectively recall memories while ignoring the vast majority of both the presenting data stream and stored information in our brains. This situation is both necessary and potentially dangerous. Too much information overwhelms decision-making capabilities, while too little risks omission of critical elements. Paralysis through analysis must be weighed against uninformed decision making. A compromise must be struck between blind adherence to preconception and rigid determination to absolute knowledge. We are obliged to do the best with what we have and can make available. That best is achieved through the ethical pursuit of truth in an environment of trust and integrity while utilizing the tools of quality management and statistical thinking. To do less is to risk lesser and perhaps harmful results. We are constantly betting that we can navigate the minefields of life with incomplete information. Integrity, both in others as well as oneself, is the minesweeper that allows us to move forward as social beings. Integrity offers the best chance for organizational enhancement in service to mission, and it is the most essential characteristic that the board should seek and demand in its CEO.

The Whole Truth

One of the greatest contributions of the legal profession to our culture is the concept of the **truth, the whole truth, and nothing but the truth**. This is widely recognized as the standard to which witnesses are sworn while providing testimony in a court of law. Interestingly, and by design, no one else in the courtroom is so duty-bound to the truth. In fact, much of legal training, most of trial preparatory efforts and courtroom actions, and a large portion of the remunerative rewards of the legal profession are geared to ensuring that only selected portions of the truth are exposed, and in many cases that the truth is overlooked either substantively or entirely. Our nation's adversarial legal system and its insinuation into our medical institutions too often sacrifices truth on the altar of self-interest and unconstrained advocacy. As Robert Kagan points out in *Adversarial Legalism*, the role of the zealous advocate is to achieve the best result for his or her client without primary regard for truth or the larger good. Adversarial cultural norms have found their way into health care boardrooms where the cooperative search for truth has been severely impeded.

An important component of the swearing in of witnesses is the acknowledgement that the "whole truth" is called for in pledging to truthful testimony. This is based upon the realization that **half-truths** can be as damaging or more damaging than lies. Because of their ability to disarm our natural lie detecting capabilities, half-truths are often more effective than lies in inducing false beliefs in targeted audiences. Directors must be on guard against half-truths and be willing to expose these representations for what they are...deliberate attempts to deceive. Half-truths represent truth decay in one of its most virulent forms.

All this is not to say that our legal system never produces justice through an adversarial search for truth. Rather, the balance is too often shifted in favor of actors on a stage who subscribe to a performative theory of truth to the exclusion of the more substantive theories of truth. Recent initiatives by the American Bar Association through its 2001 redefinition of disclosure rules are an implicit acknowledgement of the legal profession's inability to strike an acceptable ethical balance between client rights and societal interests. It is not uncommon for courtroom verdicts to run counter to public sentiments and common sense with respect to truth. By divorcing substantive theories of truth from justice we may be setting the stage for unintended consequences of a compelling nature. Boards of health care institutions need

70

to be vigilant in their efforts to avoid performative intrusions into what should be substantive commitments to truth. Skilled rhetoric should not be conflated with truthfulness. The peculiarly American tradition of adversarial legalism has little or no place in the healthcare arena where the unencumbered cooperative search for truth is called for in service to patients and mission.

Levels of Truth Ascription

The truth we seek to know is often elusive. As Oscar Wilde remarked, "The pure and simple truth is rarely pure and never simple." Part of the difficulty in seeking truth is that there exist differing levels of truth ascription to reality, each of increasing complexity:

> First order truths are those involving objects.
> Second order truths involve relationships.
> Third order truths involve processes.
> Fourth order truths deal with belief systems, the most difficult to identify and to understand.

Each of these levels of truth ascription operates throughout our daily routines. There is overlap among the four levels as well as a constant dynamic of exchange between levels during deliberations. Problems arise when we feel that we are in agreement on the basis of an accepted view at one level while major differences exist, often not consciously recognized by all parties to a process, at another level of truth ascription.

Leaders, including directors, must work to eliminate or at least minimize these unintended and sometimes deliberate discordant truth ascriptions. This can be accomplished through the balanced application of ethical **advocacy** and **inquiry**. These reflective operations, when applied consistently over time, constitute a remarkably effective means of searching for truth. Failure to recognize and expose discordant truth ascription can lead to both dysfunctional processes and unsatisfactory outcomes.

Additional attention needs to be paid to the category of implicit memories and beliefs, which operate outside of individual and group awareness. These beliefs (truths) can have profound influences on our thoughts and actions while we remain unaware of their presence. By evading consciousness these sometimes powerful influences remain undetected and out of the reach of conscious inquiry. They can at times overwhelm our working memory, which serves as the repository of mental energy and capacity from which we draw to meet the needs of process involvement. While such subconscious beliefs can be helpful and deeply ethical in nature, these beliefs can also be

71

held at significant expense and be harmful and supportive of unethical decisions and actions.

Painful Truths

There exists a broad spectrum of knowledge that is distasteful both to individuals and to organizations. This category of information includes what are known as **painful truths**. As difficult as it is to attain a truth that is agreeable, distasteful truths are dealt with by the human mind differently than is information which is perceived as either value neutral or complimentary. Human beings have developed elaborate neural networks that ease the pain of dealing with unpleasant realities. We routinely allow ourselves to see a more favorable reflection in the mirror than is warranted by the stark reality of the object being reflected.

Information and beliefs that are perceived as harmful or threatening can be a cause for **attentional anxiety**. Discomforting information is often suppressed by the mind in an effort to avoid the pain of recognition. Such repression requires constant energy input and comes at a high cost to individuals and to the institutions that they serve. There is a large body of evidence in the literature of psychology and cognitive neurosciences to support the concept of self-deception. The human mind has become accustomed to suppression of unfavorable truths. An excellent source of information regarding the psychology of self-deception is Daniel Goleman's book, *Vital Lies, Simple Truths*. While in some instances it may be necessary to suppress information for continued process involvement, across the larger spectrum of organizational endeavors such repression can exact a severe toll. Too often, when acknowledgement of the truth would hurt, the truth is simply, but often at high cost, not acknowledged.

There are several neural mechanisms for truth avoidance. These involve the concept of forgetting, and then forgetting that we have forgotten. The psychological defense mechanisms that have been described and which allow inattention to the truth include: automatism, denial, isolation, projection, rationalization, repression, reversal, selective inattention and sublimation. Taken together, these psychological defense mechanisms constitute a psychic armor that shields us from unfavorable truths about ourselves. The result is a life based in part upon self-deception. A major problem for organizations is the insinuation of such mechanisms into the activities and deliberations of directing bodies, thereby robbing the organization of useful energies and precluding truth recognition.

As this psychic armor drives us further from the truth we embrace an inaccurate view of current reality. This mistake impedes the generation of appropriate levels of creative tension, the energy that drives us towards our goals. By overestimating current capabilities we underestimate the gap between current reality and our future goals. Correspondingly, we diminish the creative energies invested in an attempt to achieve a better future. This is harmful for an individual and especially damaging for organizations at leadership levels.

Suppression of painful truths creates attentional defects referred to as lacunae. A **lacuna** is a psychological blind spot analogous to the visual blind spot present in each of our eyes. Visual lacunae serve to make part of the visual field of each eye invisible to the mind. Binocular vision allows us to overcome the blind spot in each eye by providing an overlapping visual field. This not only compensates for the blind spot in each eye, but also enhances vision by adding both a greater combined angle of vision and the dimension of depth perception. By the same token, having multiple individuals on organizational boards should allow compensation for individual psychological blind spots. However, it is often the case that the presence of multiple individuals is not effective in compensating for these blind spots. In a perverse way, groups may even expand blind spots through collusive efforts to shield their members from painful recognition of unethical behaviors.

One of the dangers inherent in the mind's ability to protect us from uncomfortable truths is the emergence of individual and group mentalities which fail to recognize what are often obvious shortcomings. Disinterested third party observers are sometimes astounded by the inability of individuals and groups to acknowledge clearly evident truths. Painful truths are repressed from individual and collective consciousness. For organizations the resultant **group think** is often a recipe for disaster. The price paid for such collective self-deception is a compromised ability to deal effectively with increasingly competitive demands. In addition, the constant and increasing requirement of energy input to support these lacunae robs the organization of resources that would be better employed in process improvement. Eventually the burden can become so great that the organization becomes trapped in a spiraling vortex of dysfunction and even organizational meltdown. Honest, sometimes brutally honest, truth-driven critical thinking is essential to a fuller understanding of process improvement and recognition of opportunities for organizational enhancement.

Groups, through shared self-deceptions, can severely inhibit the search for truth by erecting remarkably rigid psychological frames. Within these boundaries members are free to discuss concepts deemed non-threatening. Outside the frame of comfort there are notions that may be salient and even crucial, but which are not considered appropriate for discussion and consideration. Group think trumps rational inquiry. Important information and points of view are excluded. A high price is paid for this institutionalized disability to deal with reality from a foundation of truth. **Skilled incompetence**, an oxymoron introduced a generation ago by Chris Argyris, describes the situation that results from the employment of such psychological defenses by individuals and groups.

Shared self-deceptions become indirectly manifested in **protective reticence**, an unwillingness and/or inability to air controversial topics or to venture beyond organizational orthodoxy to discover truth. This thought collusion often operates outside of conscious awareness. While protective reticence may allow boards to avoid the discomfort of painful truths, this defense mechanism renders the organization more vulnerable to competitors who have a fuller grasp of reality. Shared psychological blind spots require constant and expanding energy expenditures in order to be maintained. These demands on the energies of the group can overwhelm the needs of attending to business at hand. What masquerades as a search for truth is the selected use of filtered data to support a preconceived belief. Ethical blinders can create illusions of unanimity and invulnerability where serious doubts and legitimate disagreements exist, but are precluded from surfacing.

A related concept, **cognitive dissonance**, was described over a half-century ago by Leon Festinger. This concept helps to explain the need to employ the defense mechanisms that suppress truth from our consciousness. Basically, when an individual is faced with two conflicting ideas or beliefs the more psychologically painful or threatening will be suppressed even if this means distorting or ignoring the truth. People, individually and in groups, begin to believe self-imposed lies and deceptions. As the lies are repeated, a lesson from Alice in Wonderland becomes operative. That is, if one says something three times, it must be true...the "saying is believing" phenomenon. The near-term benefit is to soothe the discomfort of a painful truth. The costs in the long run may be enormous.

As important truths are neglected or repressed, skilled incompetence becomes the modus operandi for dealing with new data and information. This may not be apparent in the short term where an individual or an organization enjoys a privileged position. It may take time for processes to manifest weakness introduced into an otherwise healthy environment, as

74

there is often a reserve of good will and resources to compensate for short-term difficulties. Unfortunately, these compensatory mechanisms, by concealing faults in truth recognition, often reinforce the willingness to believe self-deceptions, further insulating them from healthy inquiry. Ethical leadership seeks to expose these problems early in the course of their development, thereby avoiding the more difficult task of trying to uproot deceptions that have become complex and inextricably intertwined with perceptions of reality.

World history is replete with examples of such organizational psychological ploys. On a grand scale, Stalin's Soviet Union eliminated, by conservative estimates, ten to twenty million people. The horrors that befell these victims were repressed in the sanitized version of Soviet history of those times. A collective amnesia was artificially maintained regarding the atrocities. That such a large-scale collective lacuna can be made operational is testimony to the tremendous influence that these psychological ploys can exert in human affairs.

The cost of maintaining shared deceptions includes not only the inability to recognize truth and the diversion of immense psychological energies of individuals and groups from more productive endeavors, but also the emergence of an unrealistically heightened fear of acknowledgment of truth. Leadership becomes more concerned with perception than with reality. Intense mental energies and institutional resources become focused on providing positive "spins" on news that would otherwise be acknowledged for its truth content. Crafty data presentations and creative interpretations become commonplace. Style wins out over substance.

Most organizations would be immeasurably better off if ugly truths were faced head-on while focusing the collective energies of all involved on the search for root causes and fundamental solutions to problems. Individual and collective efforts are more progressively employed in preventing and correcting problems (i.e., improving quality) rather than in maintaining psychic diversions to hide painful truths (i.e., maintaining the status quo). The trade-off between acknowledging and searching for the truth on the one hand, and maintaining a distorted self-image through self-deception on the other hand, is the inability to allow truth to work to the advantage of the enterprise.

People tend to aggregate over time in such a fashion that groups share, explicitly and implicitly, a large body of self-deceptions. Whole directorships can be selected over time to conform to these deceptions. This happens through a combination of self-selection (both choosing *in* and

75

choosing *out*) through controlled nominating committee selections and voluntary or involuntary resignations. Over time an entire deliberative body can come to embrace a common pool of self-deceptions. That these individuals fail to recognize their collective faults can seriously weaken their individual and collective abilities to meet the demands of running a business. Until they recognize that they are failing to notice these defects in their beliefs, they cannot fully engage their energies in ethical pursuit of organizational improvement in service to mission. Across the organization too much energy is drained from the pool of abilities and motivation to allow optimization of process participation.

Deliberate Deceptions

Up to this point we have reviewed elements of the human psyche which operate for the most part outside of conscious awareness. Although those mechanisms impact profoundly upon the ability of individuals and groups to seek and deal with truth, they often pale in comparison to deliberate and conscious efforts to both suppress the truth and to lie.

Deliberate efforts to manipulate meaning and distort truth have become commonplace. Health care board members are often targeted for such mental manipulation, and are surprisingly susceptible to the numerous techniques of deception used to promote personal and hidden agendas. Individuals who are remarkably effective leaders in other business arenas become sitting ducks for adversarialists who use tricks of language and data manipulation to further self-serving interests at the expense of the institution which directors are by law and by ethical commitment serving in a fiduciary manner. This is in part explained (but not excused) by recognition of the honorable ends to which board members serve. However, it is dangerous to equate honorable mission with ethical process. Therein lies the rub...and the opportunity for deception.

In this section we will first explore language tricks that are employed to hide or distort truth. Then we will consider false arguments that are frequently employed to draw sought-after conclusions in the minds of the target audience. Finally the concept of 'operational definition' will be suggested as a way to drive work and deliberative processes closer to the truth and to avoid deliberate attempts to hide the truth from those who most need to know the truth.

David Nyberg, in *The Varnished Truth*, states that the English language, including gestures and facial expressions, "is bountiful in alternatives to straightforward, clear, truthful communication." Furthermore, he postulates

76

that a critical function of language is "to regulate relationships among individuals and groups...by maintaining surveillance over information revealed and concealed." According to the thesis developed in his text, deception is both a prime purpose and a fundamental property of language. Nyberg goes on to argue that what is needed is a better ability to detect lies, but that the ultimate advantage in human relationships may rest with acceptance of the status quo excepting certain egregious categories of lying. That is, we lie to ourselves and we lie to each other, and we should not fight it except in extreme cases. The latter sentiment is robustly opposed by most management theorists who write about quality and ethics.

Accepting what appear to be small lies often starts us down a slippery slope of accepting progressively more consequential distortions. Adversarialists are keenly aware of their ability to start small with respect to engaging key persons in the acceptance of marginal behaviors, often in the form of small material and psychological bribes, in anticipation of later locking these people into accepting egregious behaviors and distortions. Board members should not allow even the perception of acquiescence with unethical behaviors. The cost is too high for the organization.

Most people recognize the shortcomings of language and accept the assumption that language serves to transfer meaning from one person to another imperfectly. However, it is ethically imperative that the content of the meaning transferred should adhere as vigorously as possible to the truth. By communicating in graphic form as well as in the form of statistical process control charts (see chapter 2) the abuses that are abundant in the use of the spoken and written word are largely avoidable, provided that integrity of both data collection and data transformation are assured and that operational definitions have been established.

One of the frequent and flagrant abuses of the search for truth is the **"kill the messenger"** phenomenon. This can be carried out flagrantly or subtly, and takes the form of ad hominem attacks rather than facing the issues raised by the bearer of bad news or painful truths. This managerial style demonstrates the bankruptcy of managerial and leadership's espoused reverence for truthfulness. There are few more effective means of destroying motivation among employees than front-line knowledge that the "kill the messenger" attitude exists in the organization. Unfortunately, the prevailing culture in many organizations condones and may even encourage this type of managerial response. The lay press is replete with stories of firing whistle blowers, silencing those who disclose defects, attacking those who expose hidden agendas, and marginalizing constructive critics of the status quo. These ploys are standard fare in the "business as usual" approach to bad news. Such responses are predictable behaviors among persons trained in adversarial thinking. After all, it was adversarial thinking and tactics that allowed many of the individuals who occupy top managerial positions to have ascended to their current positions. Why turn one's back on tools and techniques that have empowered and perpetuate one's advantaged position. The fact that an individual has ascended to a top position in your organization does not prove a commitment to truthfulness. Meanwhile, lower level employees are simply not paid enough to risk truth telling in an organization where such disclosure can cost them their job or a good letter of recommendation.

The demands of health care organizational leadership in today's changing and increasingly competitive environment are too high to be met by leaders who are not fully committed to truth. Even in easier times, this leadership style did not measure up to basic ethical standards of behavior. The conduct of leadership in the face of painful truths is being held up to increasing scrutiny. Concealing or trying to define away painful truths is no longer an acceptable management style. Consumers and their representative government are holding institutions to stricter adherence to truthful reporting. Of particular interest to medical boards are the legislative initiatives under consideration to require full disclosure of adverse events to patients and patients' families. There are strong arguments for and against such mandates, but the pendulum is clearly shifting if the direction of disclosure. The tort system will have to change significantly if full disclosure is to have any chance of succeeding in its intent. Workers are similarly holding management to higher standards of dealing with the truth. A resolute commitment to truth is a common thread of the fabric of enduring world-class organizations. Such commitment should be demanded of top management by the boards of health care institutions.

There are several tricks, verbal and non-verbal, that serve the purpose of concealing or only selectively revealing parts of the truth. These ruses serve as signals to board members that they are dealing with persons of questionable commitment to truth, and include the following:

Cadence
Calculated Mumbling
Concealment
Conventions of Emphasis
Foreshortening
Gestures
Inflection
Interruption

Inverted Commas Use
Meaningfully Expressionless Expressions
Nonchalant Nodding
Pitch
Precise Miswording
Timing

All of these ploys can be used to stymie attempts to disclose the truth or to deliberately convey an understanding that deviates from the truth. The result is to transfer meanings that are distortions of what should be matters of fact. The effect may be to strip board members of their ability to exercise fiduciary responsibility.

Fallacies of Logic

Another manner in which deliberations can be driven further from the truth is in the choice of rhetorical technique used to develop arguments for or against propositions. When advocacy unduly overrides inquiry, people often resort to fallacies of logic in an effort to lend an air of legitimacy to an argument in favor of a preconceived or self-serving notion. Even in those instances wherein members of a group have been able to free the search for truth from the contamination introduced by self-deceptions and misleading communication, there remains the potential for truth decay as a result of perversions of the process of logical analysis.

As outlined by Irving Copi in *Introduction to Logic*, logic consists of the study of methods and principles used to distinguish correct from incorrect reasoning. For practical purposes, one of the most relevant categories of information that has emerged from the field of logic is that of fallacies. **Fallacies of logic** are invalid forms of argument employed to verify a conclusion. While neither truth nor falsity of a conclusion is guaranteed by the validity of an argument, the use of a fallacy of logic to support a position is an invalid means for determining truth. More often than not, conclusions arrived at through the support of fallacies of logic are suspect at best. Sometimes fallacies are used as shortcuts to conclusions that may be true. More often, fallacies are employed otherwise, namely to support statements that are not true and could not stand up to rational inquiry. Broadly speaking, there are two categories of fallacies of logic. These two categories consist of formal logical fallacies and informal logical fallacies.

Formal fallacies deal with mistakes in reasoning that evolve out of a misunderstanding or misapplication of the formal rules of deductive and inductive reasoning. These are similar to mistakes in mathematics, wherein there exist rules that must be consistently applied in order to validate the process of argument and thereby hold a conclusion to be correct. These deal with patterns of inference. This finds its parallel in the coherence theory of truth; that is, in order for the reasoning to be considered valid, the steps taken in reasoning must cohere with larger generally accepted principles. Formal fallacies constitute an important category of fallacious argument, but this is not the category of fallacy that we are most likely to encounter in daily affairs of directorship.

Informal fallacies constitute the category that is most often encountered and for which we must remain constantly on guard. As described by Douglas Walton in *Informal Logic*, these fallacies consist of errors in reasoning or deceptions that are due to improper attentiveness to the subject matter or to lack of clarity in the use of language. These forms of argument, while incorrect, can be persuasive. These fallacies often dominate deliberations where hidden agendas or self-serving goals prevail. Informal fallacies fall into two categories: fallacies of relevance and fallacies of ambiguity.

Fallacies of Relevance

The common denominator found in **fallacies of relevance** is the situation that the premise of the argument is logically irrelevant to and therefore incapable of establishing the truth of the conclusion. Among the fallacies of relevance are the following:

Ad hominem (abusive)
Ad hominem (circumstantial)
Appeal to Authority
Appeal to Force
Appeal to Pity
Appeal to Populus
Argument by Accident
Argument from Adverse Consequences
Argument from Ignorance
Begging the Question (assuming the answer)
Complex Question
Confusion of Correlation with Causation
Extended Middle
False Alternatives
False Cause
Good Person Fallacy
Half-truths (suppressed evidence)
Hasty Generalization

Inconsistency
Irrelevant Conclusion
Meaningless Question
Naturalistic Fallacy
Non-sequitur
Observational Selection
Post hoc ergo propter hoc
Special Pleading
Straw Man

All of the above mentioned fallacies of relevance share the inability to validate a truth. Many are used to gain advantage over unsuspecting or trusting individuals who would likely be much more demanding of intellectual rigor when it comes to dealing with their own business or personal finances. Occupying a position on a board of a health care institution does not relieve you of responsibilities that should under normal circumstances be in effect. This includes the responsibility to demand that such fallacies not be used to influence deliberations.

Fallacies of Ambiguity

Fallacies of ambiguity are those arguments in which the execution of the process of analysis contains unclear or ambiguous words or phrases. Meanings may change or shift subtly in the course of the development of the thought process and thereby render the process fallacious. Among the fallacies of ambiguity are the following:

Accent
Amphiboly
Composition
Division
Equivocation (literal)
Equivocation (relative)
Genetic
Weasel words

Fallacies of ambiguity can be overcome through understanding and applying the concept of **operational definition.** Popularized by W. Edwards Deming, an operational definition is a precise meaning that everyone can agree upon. Such definitions include not only strict agreements on fact, but also agreements on the processes employed to arrive at specific results. An operational definition gives communicable meaning to a concept. The term "operational definition" first appeared in *The Logic of Modern Physics* by

81

P.W. Bridgman, published in 1927. Having operational definitions of the terms used in conveying meaning to others is a crucial component of the search for truth. Such definitions can render fallacies of ambiguity nonexistent among persons cooperating ethically in the search for truth. Operational definitions can render fallacies of ambiguity non-effective when employed by adversarialists to gain advantage.

Truths Revealed, Truths Concealed

Let's now turn to a consideration of some of what is known about the human brain. Tor Norretranders, in *The User Illusion,* draws valuable insights from the cognitive neurosciences regarding human consciousness. It is estimated that at any second the awake and conscious human brain receives approximately 11 million bits of data as sensory input, about 90 percent of which is obtained through the sense of vision. Almost all of the combined sensory data input is ignored by the conscious mind. The **bandwidth of human consciousness** has been estimated to be in the range of 8-40 bits per second, and more likely at the lower end of this range. What this means is that the conscious mind can only handle a very small percentage of the sensory input. The mind relegates all but .0001 percent of awake sensory data input to subconscious levels. Even more remarkable is the ability to select what should and should not be held from consciousness, and then to shift attention to another very small segment of data input when appropriate. Continuously, the mind is able to shift attention rapidly and seamlessly to appropriate inputs from among the millions of data bits available. The ability to allocate this tiny bandwidth of consciousness is essential to optimal functioning. To have this small but crucial bandwidth contaminated by input in service to hidden agendas borders on criminal seizure of a precious commodity. Trustworthiness and integrity help to assure the availability of this resource for the good of the order.

Along a similar line of understanding brain function, there exists the concept of **working memory**. Working memory represents the attention capability of the mind and describes the number of conscious thoughts that we can bring to bear on a task before us. Working memory, as described by George A. Miller in 1956, has a limit estimated to be 7 plus or minus 2. That is, we can hold in present awareness only 5 to 9 ideas or symbols as we navigate the challenges of problem solving. This means that many, if not a majority, of pertinent ideas are of necessity not able to be consciously brought to bear on a task before us. Remarkably, the mind is able to consistently select the few most pertinent thoughts to bear on the issue at hand. To have working memory contaminated by lies and deceptions can be lethally destructive of the capacity to seek truth. This limitation of individual ability underscores the potential for a group to be less likely to omit relevant facts from deliberation. As we have seen, however, group psychodynamics may work to restrict even further the number of items available for consideration through mechanisms of shared psychic armor as manifest in skilled incompetence and protective reticence.

Given the rather severe limitations placed upon us by our biology, we need to make truth recognition more readily attainable. As pointed out by Daniel Dennett in *Consciousness Explained*: "...the techniques of (computer) graphics...permit huge arrays of data to be presented in a format that lets the superb pattern recognition capabilities of human vision ...keep track of what is relevant, and remind us to ask the right questions at the right times." When data are transformed into graphic form hidden meanings or the lack thereof are more readily apparent.

From the body of knowledge known as quality management some remarkably effective means of data interpretation have been made available. In particular, the emphasis upon graphic presentation of data is considered central to communicating truth. While this concept is more fully developed in chapter 2, it should be noted that straightforward graphs and charts can summarize reams of data that are often, and not infrequently by design, impenetrable. Of special interest are Statistical Process Control Charts (SPC charts). These charts display appropriate data and data subgroups over time and thereby show a much clearer picture of current reality and trends in performance. The advantage to such reporting is that the limited capacities of working memory and conscious sensory input can be more efficaciously employed. Painful truths can be expressed. However, the effectiveness of this approach is sensitively dependent upon the integrity of both data collection and data transformation.

Data entry is one of the newly found leverage points that unethical people have discovered in health care institutions. For a relatively small price, data entry can be manipulated to allow distortions and lies to emerge from the process of statistical analysis. In an era of self-reporting, there are no limits to which data mining, data suppression, and data manufacturing can be carried on in service to hidden agendas. Integrity is the insurance policy that the board holds to assure the accuracy and appropriateness of data entry. The people who control data entry are increasingly able to manipulate perceptions of reality upon which decisions rest. These are key players in the internal politics of your institution. Increasingly they are key players in external affairs as well. You cannot afford to take data at face value. It is incumbent upon board members to understand the methodology of data collection and transformation prior to making important decisions.

The simple principles outlined in this chapter can spell the difference between life and death. A spectacular example of the failure to apply ethical principles in the pursuit of truth was the Challenger space shuttle disaster of January 28, 1986. This was an entirely avoidable catastrophe. Two engineers had strongly objected to the launch in cold weather on the grounds of O-ring test failures at low temperatures. Their warnings were not passed along to higher levels as there were political pressures to not delay the launch. A group think mentality of protective reticence prevailed. Vital truths had been kept from collective awareness. Later, after testifying at the inquiry these two engineers were demoted, only to be reinstated after public outcry. The "kill the messenger" mentality had emerged. Furthermore, while the engineers had known of the O-ring problems, they had not shown the data in a compelling way. A simple data conversion to a graphic presentation could have convinced those who were in positions of authority to postpone the launch.

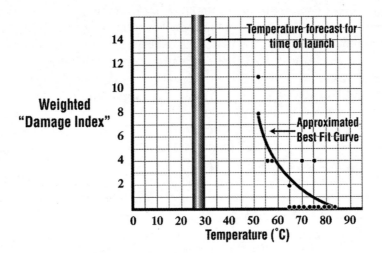

As presented by Ivan Valiela in *Doing Science*, the plot of damage index vs. temperature would have made it clear to those involved that to launch at so low a temperature was begging for disaster.

Two fundamental principles were violated. First, the messengers were marginalized and eventually punished for their truthfulness. Second, the data were not made available in a format easily accessible to non-engineers. Ethical behavior would have prevented the silencing of the concerns of the engineers. Understanding the limitations of the human mind to interpret data and the improved ability to recognize information in graphic form would have made it clear to others that the danger was real and significant.

The situation is not very different in many health care institutions. Truths are often not allowed to surface, and clear dangers are often buried in data banks. Board members need to force open the issue of truthful reporting and insist upon clarity and comprehensibility in data presentation. Lives may hang in the balance.

Ethical management demands a concerted effort to search for, recognize, communicate, and act upon the truth. This respect for truth must operate fully among all stakeholders. Reverence for unadulterated truth is a requirement of the health care field unlike any other arena of human endeavor. People's lives are literally dependent upon this principle of behavior. You should not underestimate the pervasive effects that occur when truth avoidance and manipulated meanings exist at the highest levels of institutional leadership. The result is often a proliferation of dysfunctional process involvement that works its way throughout the organization and ultimately adversely impacts patient care. As a board member you must realize that you hold the lives of people, often friends and relatives, in your hands. The whole truth you seek can help them greatly; truth suppressed or avoided can cause irreparable harm. Many people in positions of board service are provided a Potemkin-village view of the front-line workings of their organization. When they present in need of services, board members and their families often receive VIP treatment reserved for a very few, belying the problems facing health care consumers on a daily basis. Others in positions of privilege simply seek services elsewhere for themselves and their families rather than deal with the unpleasant truths of their own facilities.

Ethical management places a heavy emphasis on truth and the honest search for truth. Truth is the foundation upon which all human efforts to improve are built. If this platform is not based on an accurate understanding of reality, then there is little chance that individual or group efforts will continuously or optimally improve. Truth telling, as described by J.L.Mackie in *Ethics: Inventing Right and Wrong*, "...naturally goes along with cooperation; it is not obviously reasonable to tell the truth to a competitor or to an enemy." While Mackie is addressing the idea of enduring ethical standards, he also hits upon a critical distinction between cooperative and adversarial cultures. The importance of organizational culture is more fully discussed in chapter 1, so only a brief summary is included here.

In the **adversarial cultural paradigm**, individuals and groups view reality as consisting of a fixed or shrinking pie of opportunity. Each person gets his or her slice at the expense of another. The 'you vs. me' and 'us vs. them' mentalities prevail as every encounter is viewed as a potential win-lose situation. The adversarial cultural paradigm has come to prevail in our market economy. In health care it has also become the predominant mindset pitting individuals and institutions at odds with each other. Alternatively, there exists a **cooperative cultural paradigm** wherein reality is viewed as consisting of a growing pie of opportunity. People operating under the cooperative belief system feel that each person or group can achieve more with a lesser percentage slice of an increasingly larger pie. Teamwork is the operative strategy and win-win scenarios are the norm. This is not the prevailing expectation in our economy today. It was a more widespread persuasion in health care, particularly in the non-profit sector, in the past.

In the cooperative paradigm the belief in potential to grow the pie is central. In the adversarial paradigm the potential for growth of the commons is replaced by preoccupation with self-service. As the concept of improving the good of the order is removed from the working memory of adversarialists, the idea of a shrinking pie of opportunity becomes a self-fulfilling prophesy. The cooperative ethic remains ideally suited to the ethical governance of health care institutions. Health care is currently trapped in a vortex of adversarial reliance upon increasingly legalistic operations which, in turn, reinforces and drives the sector further into the adversarial cultural milieu. This state of affairs is not healthy for the sector over the long term, and it is detrimental to individual institutions here and now.

In an adversarial culture, everyone is a real or potential enemy. Many of those who gather at the table for board deliberations will be perceived as threats to the status quo and adversarial agendas. As a result, even at the board level of institutional stewardship the search for truth will be impaled upon the bayonets of self-interest.

Trust

Trust according to a dictionary definition includes " assured reliance on the character, ability, strength or truth of someone or something." To be trustworthy is to possess both the ability and willingness to perform or deliver at or above the level promised. It is the combination of capability and reliability (i.e. trustworthiness) of institutional directorship and executive leadership that leads to trust throughout the organization. In the health care field, consumers place their lives in the hands of providers, both people and institutions, whom they deem to be trustworthy. Employees willingly invest discretionary efforts in the search for truth and organizational enhancement when, and only when, they perceive that an atmosphere of trust envelops

86

their interactions with others. Absent trust the engine of truth sputters to a halt. Trust is absolutely necessary for meaningful continuous improvement.

Trust is not easily gained. Humans, being social animals, have evolved a rather elaborate neural network to detect people and representations that are not trustworthy. The survival of early hunter-gatherers was very sensitive to being able to discern in others the reliable from the unreliable. Any group that developed dependable neural mechanisms for truth and trust detection surely was afforded a survival advantage. Such neural networks, however far they may be from being understood, play a critical role in social progress.

Modern societies have witnessed the emergence of professions whose goal is to disarm and confuse this human trait, often in order to gain positional or financial advantage. Perhaps the most recent field to have been invaded by this cadre of truth-trumpers and spin-meisters has been health care. When health care constituted only a small portion of the GDP the field was pretty much left to its own devices for regulating the application of virtues to the workplace. With the rapid growth in money available to the health care economy following the introduction of Medicare legislation in 1965 (and which will soon reach $2 trillion per year in the United States), the field of health care has become too financially attractive to escape the attention of resourceful people from all walks of life. Dishonorable people willing to place self-service above institutional well-being come in all shapes and sizes. Some may be present at your board meetings, in your executive suite, or in overpriced consultative positions. You need to ferret out these people in order to protect the integrity of institutional improvement in service to mission.

As cited by Matt Ridley in *The Origins of Virtue*, an honest individual values trustworthiness for its own sake. Material reward for trustworthiness is not a consideration and the honest person can be trusted where his behavior cannot be monitored. This virtue creates valuable opportunities as "Trust is a form of social capital as money is a form of actual capital...It pays dividends in the currency of more trust." Perhaps of most importance in service to mission is that trust allows truth to be spoken, heard, and acted upon.

Trust has been referred to as the highest form of human motivation. It enables the application of intense levels of discretionary efforts on behalf of institutional objectives. Trust is the fuel that powers the engine of learning in pursuit of truth. Except in situations wherein the aura of a position held can elicit trust (and there are fewer and fewer such trust havens existing in our increasingly cynical and multicultural society) it takes time and effort to build trust. Trust can be destroyed in an instant. Trust represents a deep emotional as well as intellectual investment in another. Violation of trust scars deeply and in some cases irrevocably.

There is a special obligation to be trustworthy for those who choose to serve on boards of health care organizations. In addition to the compelling ethical obligations that the assumption of such service entails, there is a clear legal obligation of **fiduciary responsibility**. According to *Black's Law Dictionary*, a person holding the position of trustee by his own undertaking must "...with scrupulous good faith and candor ..." act on behalf of the organization and not on one's own behalf. This obligation includes prohibition against investing the money or property in anything speculative or imprudent. Further, the embezzlement or misappropriation of trust funds or endowment monies held in a fiduciary manner constitutes **defalcation**. The concept of trust is one area where there exists a deep concordance between the spirit of the law and ethical behavior.

An excellent synopsis of the concept of trust as a virtue is provided by Stephen Covey in *The 7 Habits of Highly Effective People*. Covey likens the building of trust to an emotional bank account that requires specific and sustained deposits. These deposits include:

Understanding the Individual
Attending to Little Things
Keeping Commitments
Clarifying Expectations
Showing Personal Integrity
Apologizing Sincerely When you Make a Withdrawal

These six elements constitute necessary components for building effective interdependent relationships. All are required in an effort to build and maintain trust. Trust, in turn, allows process improvement to continue at optimal levels through the voluntary commitment of truthful energies and enthusiasm.

In summary, building trust requires that one deal with others in a manner that consistently demonstrates a level of respect for others that one would chose for oneself. Germane to this point is the willingness to remain faithful to those who are not present. By defending the position and character of those who are not present, those who are present gain a heightened respect for the character of leadership and an increased willingness to invest their trust in that leadership. Boards need to be skeptical of those who choose to disparage the character and commitments of others or to represent the opinions of others when those others are not present to respond. In the case of ad hominem attacks, it is likely that the object of the criticism will never be made fully aware of the harmful claims. Corrupt leadership depends upon and can often count on the protective reticence of the board.

Trust is the virtue that enables truth to be fully revealed and accurately reported. It serves as the fuel that powers the engine of truth. In turn, both trustworthiness and truthfulness are essential components of integrity.

Integrity

By far the most important concept of this most important chapter, **integrity** is the linchpin of ethical behavior. Integrity is a metavirtue, both deriving from the proper alignment of virtues and serving as an overarching descriptor of consistently virtuous behavior. A state of integrity is exceedingly difficult to attain and maintain both for individuals and for organizations. At an organizational level, integrity requires constant vigilance by the board. Absent integrity there is little that an organization can do to optimize institutional performance because the absence of integrity precludes the full engagement the discretionary efforts of stakeholders in furtherance of the institutional mission.

Almost no organization would omit integrity from its list of core values in today's regulatory environment. Core values have become standard fare for both in-house and public consumption, not because administrators have become more attuned to the need for ethical underpinnings, but because reviewing bodies such as the JCAHO have, through adaptations of quality management theories, made it a requirement that organizations document ongoing attempts to meet minimal ethical standards. These standards are often met by paying lip service to a list of values that have come to include an almost obligatory reference to integrity.

At many institutions professing a commitment to integrity, the hypocrisy of the declaration of core values is readily apparent to front-line workers. Humans are remarkably adept at detecting a mismatch between words and actions. The failure of institutional leadership to "walk the talk" of integrity becomes a standing joke among insiders, adversely affecting interactions at all levels and ultimately negatively impacting patient care. Too often, executives and board members lack a working knowledge of the definition of integrity, and too few are willing to insist that integrity be a guiding principle for their organization.

Integrity reveals itself not so much as a sense of right and wrong but rather as the faculty that allows us to discern the truth of right and wrong and to consistently act in an ethically forthright manner even when doing so is to one's disadvantage. Integrity is reflected in the willingness to keep ethical commitments in the face of adversity when there is an easier or even financially more attractive way to avoid such commitments. Integrity is the foundation principle upon which trust is established. Integrity is the keystone of the arch of human decency under which effective human relationships are nurtured.

Ethical flaws in the fabric of an institution are quick to attract cheaters and deceivers who are constantly on the lookout for opportunities to advance personal agendas at the expense of the order. Like maggots, they are looking for the easy meal (wealth transfer rather than wealth creation) at the trough of accumulated public trust and unprotected goodwill. Rents in the fabric of integrity are easily exploited and expanded. The process of degradation of the ethical fabric of the institution, if left to its own devices, becomes increasingly difficult to halt and reverse. In a process that is reminiscent of the Lemons Principle in economic theory (wherein the bad drives out the good), unethical people drive out honorable people in the organization.

As discussed by Stephen L. Carter in *(integrity)*, there are four elements which taken together suggest the existence of a state of integrity. Board members should be familiar with all four elements and demand these of themselves and of their executive staff. All four elements must be operative for integrity to hold for an individual. More importantly and with more difficulty, for a health care institution to exhibit integrity these four essential elements must be evidenced throughout the organization, both in its vertical and horizontal extensions and across time.

Integrity

1. A keen sense of right and wrong and the ability to discern the difference.
2. The ability and willingness to speak openly to the distinction between right and wrong even when and where expression of such views is unpopular.
3. The willingness to act on the distinction, even at personal cost.
4. Consistent application of elements 1, 2, and 3 over time and without exception. For persons in positions of fiduciary responsibility, this means to demand unwavering adherence to these elements by administrative and executive staff.

Given the straightforward description of the elements of integrity and the stringent requirements that they entail, it is clear that many of our health care

90

institutions fail to satisfy this most fundamental of ethical principles. The failure to measure up will exact a demanding toll on the organization over time, rendering the institution vulnerable to failure and takeover (both from within and without), and ultimately to surrender of its mission. Integrity serves to disdain short-term expediency in favor of long term prudence, an approach to decision-making that best serves the institution's ability to survive and thrive over time.

Boards have an individual and collective tendency to fail to acknowledge their responsibility to assure adherence to strict ethical standards. There are widespread feelings that such ethical oversight is not a necessary requirement of board service, that to bring up such concerns is an inappropriate use of board time, and that ethical distinctions, other than those hot button issues such as sexual harassment, are best left to the discretion of the CEO and administrative staff. The executive and administrative staff, in turn, are usually happy to not be held accountable to the board for such concerns. The result is often a carte blanche for the administration to freely interpret for the board the moral dimensions of decisions and actions wherein the ethical dimensions of process involvement are most often disregarded and almost all attention is diverted to short-term financial outcomes. The danger inherent in this state of affairs was captured by Albert Einstein: "Momentary success carries more power of conviction for most people than reflections on principle."

Furthermore, board members should be aware that there are two levels at which integrity functions: personal and professional. At the professional level, integrity requires the assumption of prior ethical commitments as well as rejection of unethical debts incurred through the position that is freely accepted. To fail to deliver on those prior ethical commitments is a declaration of lack of institutional integrity. To perpetuate dishonorable deals speaks loudly to intent to continue business as usual. This scenario constitutes a hackneyed trick employed by unethical boards to absolve themselves of debts accrued by former directors and executives. The usual mantra goes something like this: "I know that the last CEO/director was a person who did bad things and made promises he didn't keep. However, I'm different. Let's wipe the slate clean and start over." This perpetuates a cycle of unethical behaviors to which no one is held accountable as the new CEO/director will sooner or later be replaced and any newly accrued debts will again ask to be forgiven in this never ending story. The lesson learned is to embolden adversarialists in their unethical behaviors as the likelihood is high that they will have their debts expunged with the next round of leadership in the executive office. As a board member you must not fall for this rationalization. Front-line workers easily see through this charade.

An additional pitfall that you need to avoid is that of assuming that the practices of a person occupying an elevated role are ethically correct simply because that individual has ascended to a high level along the organizational chart. Roles do not grant ethical permissions to perform acts that would otherwise be deemed unacceptable. There is nothing inherent in the role of board membership or chairmanship or the position of president or CEO that allows one to overwrite what would otherwise be recognized as ethical constraints. As aptly put by Arthur Applbaum in *Ethics for Adversaries*, "Institutions and the roles they create cannot mint moral permissions to do what otherwise would be morally prohibited." This is a lesson clear to many who are far less formally educated than those who have managed to attain positions of influence in health care organizations. It is only sophisticated sophistry that supports, through arguments revealed earlier in this chapter, the granting of privileges outside the domain of integrity, truth, and trust. You cannot allow your executives and officers to assume a position of moral non-accountability on the basis of the role that they occupy. You must hold yourself and fellow board members to standards of integrity commensurate with the responsibilities of the public and private trust you have assumed. You have both legal and moral obligation to insure against the unethical abuse of authority and by so doing to better promote the mission of the institution that you have agreed to serve

The field of organizational behavior has evolved to a fuller understanding of human behavior and the central role that integrity holds in the value matrix against which actions are judged. As described by Stephen P. Robbins in *Essentials of Organizational Behavior*, enhanced understanding has led to theories of equity and expectancy that best define what motivates people. Highly motivated employees bring commitment to the workplace. An organization cannot purchase commitment from its workforce. The respect of employees must be earned through a clearly and consistently demonstrated respect for truth, an unshakable dedication to trust, and unflinching integrity.

The dangers inherent in the failure to maintain integrity amount to the failure to understand human behavior. No organization can long survive with leadership that fails to act in accordance with this basic principle. The problem of lack of integrity lies at the root of many if not most of the failures of health care institutions, and often is the operative shortcoming in those that are experiencing the throes of marginal survival in an increasingly challenging health care environment. If your institution lacks integrity you need read no further. All of the information contained in the remainder of this chapter and in all other chapters of this book cannot stave off failure if your organization, starting with your board, lacks integrity. To be sure, integrity alone will not guarantee your organization's success. However, integrity is the most valuable attribute that you bring to the table in service to your institutional mission.

The Learning Ladder

Human learning begins with data reception, progresses through steps of information, knowledge, and understanding, and ultimately matures to wisdom. Successively, at each of the steps there should be a fuller and more applicable grasp of reality (i.e. truth) enabling the individual to deal more effectively with problems, improve process performance, and ultimately enhance outcomes.

For a group of persons, such as a board of directors, the same sequence also pertains. However, for a group or organization the pitfalls along the way are far more numerous as there are more portals of data input and more handoffs along the information stream wherein deviations from the truth can occur. As more persons become involved and more levels of reporting are required, not only are the potential opportunities for truth decay multiplied, but time itself can intervene to render the data less relevant to the situation existing by the time decisions are made and changes implemented.

Schematically, and in the emotion-free language of statistical thinking, the pursuit of truth can be envisioned as the passage along a continuum through the stages:

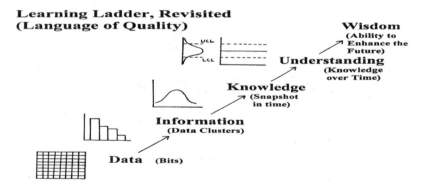

Attaining wisdom represents the ideal to which leadership should strive in the deliberative processes that come before the organization. While wisdom is at best difficult to achieve, it is the one dimension of the learning ladder that most people implicitly believe they have attained. Acting from an unwise assumption of the possession of wisdom, people too often make major decisions on the basis of data presentations alone. Oftentimes there is no recognition of the need to drive the learning process along the continuum of enhanced understanding before committing institutional resources (in the case of non-profits, public resources), to projects only incompletely understood.

Alternatively, this schematic can be viewed as a serial transfer of truth throughout an organization from the front line through the levels of administration and ultimately to the board. At each level the completeness and authenticity of the data and its transformation are highly dependent on an envelope of trust in an atmosphere of integrity. Absent trust and integrity the tendency is to distort the truth by any combination of fabrication, falsification, selective inclusion and exclusion, or plagiarism of data. The usual result is to pass along good news and to suppress bad news at each step of the reporting process. This tendency derives from the perceived need to look good in the eyes of one's superiors, a prevalent inclination in an organization lacking a culture of trust and integrity. By the time important truths should have reached top levels of the organizational chart they have often been totally suppressed or so substantively altered that the picture presented bears little resemblance to reality. This situation can arise for any of numerous reasons discussed in the section on truth as well as lack of understanding and application of principles of data transformation discussed in chapter 2. Whether intentional or inadvertent, the organization is not well served by the decomposition of truth, and the ability to fulfill mission suffers.

There is no more important function for a board of a health care institution than to assure that organizational leadership is behaving ethically. Insisting upon ethical behavior is the most important step that the directorship can take to drive the search for truth as fully and accurately as possible. The unencumbered search for truth is critically and sensitively dependent upon trust and integrity.

Summary

Ethical management has no more natural fit in any province of endeavor than in the health care field. The reality in today's health care economy is that ethical leadership has taken a back seat to more traditional styles of adversarial behaviors at all levels of leadership, including boards of directors. Too many directors and trustees have abdicated their responsibility to assure that ethical principles prevail in the institutions they oversee. In part this is the result of conflating honorable ends declared in the

94

mission statement with the oftentimes dishonorable means employed by management and trustees in furtherance of personal or hidden agendas.

Among health care and related institutions, the entire spectrum ranging from small hospitals to huge medical conglomerates have fallen prey to unscrupulous individuals. Con men have found in the health care field accumulated wealth measuring in the billions of dollars that is available to those who have learned the modern lesson that there is more easy money to be gained through unethical wealth transfer than honorable wealth creation. Witness the Allegheney Health System debacle of the 1990s wherein hundreds of millions of dollars of institutional endowments disappeared across the state of Pennsylvania. Ultimately, the public bears the expense of non-profit institutional dysfunction and failure when boards fail to insist that both they themselves and the management of their organizations adhere to ethical principles of behavior. Effectively, the end result amounts to abdication of fiduciary responsibility. This also happens to be illegal.

Ethical management places a heavy emphasis on the unadulterated search for truth. Truth, in turn, provides the foundation from which quality improvement proceeds. If this foundation is not firmly based on an accurate understanding of reality by all stakeholders, then there is little chance that an individual or organization can continuously improve, and the doors are opened to perpetrators of fraud and abuse.

Individuals and institutions which, through self-deception or deliberate suppression of the truth, believe that they are better than they are will see little need for the investment of appropriate resources to improve current conditions. The result is insufficient creative tension and under-investment in process improvement. While a few highly-positioned adversarialists may profit handsomely through inflated compensation packages and golden parachutes, the vast majority in the organization will bear the burdens imposed unnecessarily by the incurred failures to achieve established organizational goals. On the flip side, if an individual or group perceives itself to be worse than they are, then an over-investment of resources that could be better employed in an alternative process may ensue.

It is not an uncommon strategy for consultants and senior administrators to play both sides of the deception fence. By overstating existing problems among the front-line workforce (i.e. overstaffed and under motivated) they set themselves up to look good and justify exorbitant salaries and consultative fees by recommending cuts in the ranks of those who are not the cause of institutional problems. These same consultants and administrators offer false praise to the board for the board's role in governance and insight in having hired them, playing on the inability and/or unwillingness of directors to face the painful truths of substandard stewardship.

Some consultants and CEOs spend more time and effort honing their wily skills than in identifying root causes of problems and recommending fundamental solutions. They stroke the egos of those in positions of higher authority (the real source of most major problems) and in so doing render the board even less capable of truth recognition. This situation ultimately robs the institution of better resource allocation and lessens the likelihood of optimization of service to mission. One highly paid consultant told me that he was not hired to solve problems. Rather, his job was to balance the budget in the short term. When the illogic of ignoring real problems by sweeping them under a synthetic carpet of short-term financial improvement was pointed out, this consultant responded that it was not uncommon to have institutions hire his firm back after two or three years to reevaluate a situation that was likely to have reverted to even deeper distress. Board members should recognize this con game for what it is.

A useful way to view the role of board leadership is to think of the substantive theories of truth in the form of a Venn diagram. The three theories, taken together, help leadership to arrive at an operational concept of truth. The correspondence theory assures the integrity of data collection and entry and understanding of current reality. The coherence theory comes into play in both the application of principles of statistics to data transformation along the learning ladder and in using the language of statistics to eliminate the pitfalls inherent in the use and misuse of written and spoken language. The pragmatic theory with its concern for usefulness helps to drive home the centrality of customer satisfaction and outcome assessment. Taken together, the concept looks like this:

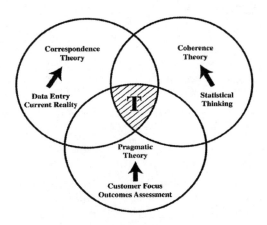

When the directorship of an organization understands and commits to the centrality of truth **(T)** the stage is set for transformational leadership and world-class performance in service to mission. The strength of the scientific method of inquiry rests in large part upon the search for the central truth **(T)** as depicted in this illustration.

However, truthfulness alone will not guarantee institutional success. Both trust and integrity must also be a part of organizational culture. Truth serves as the engine that drives progress. Trust is the fuel that allows the whole truth to transfer across organizational and functional boundaries and thereby foster progress through continuous improvement. Integrity, by nurturing the emergence of trust, provides the atmosphere essential to progress. Integrity also assures that data at the entry level is both valid and appropriate.

The learning ladder then takes on a new appearance that places an emphasis on ethical principles.

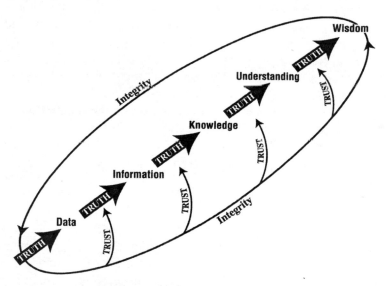

A simple but remarkably effective test to determine if a decision is ethical is provided by Kenneth Blanchard and Norman Vincent Peale in *The Power of Ethical Management*. This test consists of three **"ethics check questions:"**

1. Is it **legal**…does it violate either civil law or organizational policy?
2. Is it **balanced**…is it fair to all stakeholders in both short and long term?

3. How will I feel about myself if my decision were made public and if my family knew about it...will I be **proud** of myself?

Any answer less than an unequivocal yes to all three of the above questions strongly suggests that at best your decision rests on shaky ethical grounds and should be revisited. More likely this means that the choice or action you are contemplating is unethical and ultimately not in the best interests of your organization. This simple checklist would expose the vast majority of unethical considerations prior to their implementation.

The value of ethical behavior extends far beyond the immediacy of time, place, and the parties to a decision. Very few unethical behaviors have as their primary incentive the destruction of the institution. Most often, unethical actions are taken to advance narrow, selfish, short-term agendas. However, unethical behaviors lie at the root of the long-term failure of many health care organizations. The reason that this scenario of failure plays out lies in the importance of both secondary effects and externalities. Secondary effects are those effects on the parties to a decision that are not anticipated to be primary outcomes of the transaction. Externalities are consequences that occur to individuals or organizations that rest outside of the system of deliberation. Secondary effects and externalities together contribute to the category of **unintended consequences**. While unintended consequences are usually removed in time, place, and person from the initial transaction, they often exert profound influences in determining the ultimate outcomes of decisions. As noted by Matt Ridley in *The Origins of Virtue*, ethical sentiments "... are problem-solving devices designed to make highly social creatures effective at ...settling the conflict between short-term expediency and long-term prudence in favor of the latter."

Ethical underpinnings to process involvement provide the best protection against adverse unintended consequences. Additionally, the ethical pursuit of truth renders working memory and the limited bandwidth of consciousness as effective as possible in service to mission. These are the reasons that human societies have evolved to so highly value truthfulness, trustworthiness, and integrity. Much of the havoc that has been wreaked on health care and related institutions could have been avoided by the consistent application of this straightforward ethics checklist by board members and CEOs. For you and the future of your institution it is imperative that you dedicate yourself to the personal and professional application of the principles of truth, trust, and integrity. No less is acceptable of health care board members who are stewards of the public trust.

NOTES:

99

NOTES:

100

Chapter 5

Health Care Fraud
Truth, Justice and the "New" American Way

A Primer on fraud and antitrust issues for health care providers

James M. Sysko, S.T.B., M.S., J.D.

Issues of law have become so pervasive in the practice of modern medicine that the health care practitioner often needs a manual to understand principles and fundamentals of that law. He or she may also require daily access to the Internet in order to stay abreast of developments related to statutes, regulations, and their interpretation and application by the courts and administrative agencies. Casual conversations may focus on the latest malpractice verdict, legislative efforts for tort reform, or the socio-economic struggle for a patients' "bill of rights". Some specialists, more conversant in health law, may often speak in "code" using such acronyms as "ERISA", "EMTALA" or "COBRA" when addressing a matter of "medical" interest or concern.

This brief presentation is intended to offer the reader an overview of two categories of health care law which, while often complex, are truly intended to deal with issues of fundamental fairness. The areas of health care fraud and antitrust law are elaborate and somewhat convoluted mechanisms which hypothetically extol the virtues of honesty and equity. Unfortunately, our parents' encouragement to simply "do the right thing" becomes difficult advice to follow when one feels like "Alice" entering the "Wonderland" of health care law.

Fraud and Abuse

Common Law Fraud

In order to better understand the intricacies of laws and regulations dealing with health care fraud and abuse, one must first appreciate the distinction between the relative simplicity of "common law" fraud and the daunting complexity of its modern statutory counterparts. People have lied and cheated for time immemorial. The courts in the Anglo-American system of justice have developed a "test" or "standard" for determining whether one has committed a fraud against another. This test has become known as the "common law fraud" standard and is generally considered to consist of five elements which must be established in order to prove that a fraud has, in fact, been perpetrated.

The five elements are sequentially as follows:

1) A lie or deception;
2) Knowledge of the lie or deception (e.g. not a mistake);
3) Reliance by another party on that lie or deception;
4) A detriment or harm resulting from that reliance;
5) Damages suffered as a result of the detrimental reliance on the lie.

Although this standard is still utilized by the courts in various contexts, the rather heavy burden of proof it places on the plaintiff or the prosecutor has been supplanted by the more succinct standards of statutory fraud which have been created by Congress, the state legislatures and their administrative agencies in an effort to combat the estimated $100 billion in annual losses to health care fraud.

The Statutory Scheme

A myriad of rules and regulations have been promulgated, primarily by the Federal government, in response to clever scams, staggering losses and the all too pervasive goal of many citizens and/or organizations to "beat the system". As a society, Americans seem to be more tolerant of crimes committed with pens than they are of crimes committed with guns. Cheating on taxes, defrauding insurance companies and keeping "two sets of books" have created a "gray" if not a "black" market mentality among some people who see no harm resulting from, or victim of, their deceptive practices. Understandably, the government has reacted--some would say overreacted-- with a host of rules and regulations to safeguard the integrity of the "system" under assault.

False Claims

Notwithstanding the checks and balances built into the Medicare and Medicaid payment programs, those programs trust and depend upon the providers to ensure the accuracy and integrity of the claims submitted for payment. The intentional misrepresentation of facts and figures to Medicare or Medicaid will subject the provider to prosecution on felony charges of health care fraud. Even "innocent" errors may expose the provider to liability for thousands of dollars in civil penalties and/or repayment.

Common violations include providers billing for services not performed or billing for services "performed" on deceased patients. Of particular concern is the all too prevalent practice of "upcoding" a reimbursement claim in order to obtain a higher payment from the government. The practice is widespread as a result of the providers' rationalization wherein a justification for the over-billing will be arrived at as a result of the perception that the programs' reimbursement rates are either inadequate or that the government is really not a "victim." Needless to say, these justifications for the submission of a false claim will carry no weight with prosecutors and could result in disastrous consequences for the individual or organization including substantial fines, restitution and even imprisonment.

In December, 2000, HCA-The Healthcare Co., the nation's largest for profit hospital chain, pleaded guilty to defrauding government health care programs and agreed to pay more than $840 million in fines, civil penalties and damages. The company was accused of over-billing the government for services it performed, charging for services it did not perform and for submitting bills that were not eligible for reimbursement. Additionally, fraud and abuse were considered so widespread in the home health industry that President Clinton imposed a moratorium on the licensing of new home health care agencies until "corrections" could be made. The gravity of the problem and the severity of the government's response were summarized by then Attorney General Janet Reno who in 2000 said, "Health care fraud impacts every American citizen. If you over-bill the U.S. taxpayer, then we are going to make you pay it back and then some." Clearly, the government does not consider the submission of false claims a "victimless" crime.

Kickbacks

Although usually associated with organized crime or corrupt politicians, kickbacks have emerged as an area of grave concern for the administrators of the Medicare and Medicaid programs. The law prohibits one from giving or receiving anything of value to induce the referral of a Medicare or Medicaid patient or to induce the purchase of goods or services subject to reimbursement by the programs. The prohibitions cover both direct and indirect as well as overt or covert remuneration.

Turning to the traditional understanding of kickbacks and the common law fraud doctrine, providers initially believed that the intent of the parties would serve as the determining factor for establishing criminal misconduct. The government quickly rejected this interpretation citing the subjectivity of determining intent and the complexity of many of the business relationships in which kickbacks may play a role.

Providers then attempted to fashion a compromise in which the payment of inducements would be prosecuted only if the *sole* purpose of the payment was to induce referrals. This compromise was offered in recognition of special situations in which some referrals may be an indirect result of an inducement or incentive in another business relationship such as when rural hospitals would benefit indirectly from programs to attract physicians to their market. Again, regulators rejected the standard citing vagueness and subjectivity.

Prosecutors and regulators would accept nothing less than an absolute ban on kickbacks wherein the giving or receiving of anything of value in exchange for a referral, intentional or unintentional, direct or indirect, would be considered actionable under the law. This absolutist approach resulted in cynicism and criticism by the providers so widespread that Congress directed the Office of Inspector General of the Department of Health and Human Services to issue advisory opinions to providers as part of the Health Insurance Portability and Accountability Act of 1996. Those advisory opinions are available on the OIG's web site and are intended to assist providers with good faith compliance with the law.

Self-Referrals

In the mid-1980s, regulators recognized an emerging and troubling trend in which physicians were engaged in the practice of referring patients to ancillary health care facilities in which the physicians or their family members had a financial stake. The practice was deemed unacceptable due to the perceived conflict of interest and the likelihood that dubious referrals would increase the overall cost of health care.

The problem was first addressed in 1989 when Congressman Peter Stark of California sponsored legislation that would prohibit physicians from referring patients to clinical laboratories in which the physician or an immediate family member had a financial interest. The statute prohibited the billing for such a referral to Medicare or any third party payer for services rendered pursuant to a prohibited referral. Although limited exceptions to the rule were created, the effect was to create a firewall between the physician and clinical laboratory services.

Congress revisited this arena of perceived and actual physician conflicts of interest in 1993 when it extended the payment prohibitions to Medicaid billings and included the additional health care services of physical and occupational therapy, radiology services, radiation therapy, durable medical equipment, home health services, and inpatient and outpatient hospital services, *inter alia*. These new areas of "coverage" became commonly known as the "Stark II" laws.

Although the laws do not categorically prohibit all physician or physician family interests in the ownership of health care facilities or ancillary operations, they make such ownership interests difficult or impractical by preventing reimbursement for a broad range of prohibited referrals. The Healthcare Finance Administration has created a maze of definitions and exceptions to the prohibitions which have had the effect of confusing practitioners, enriching lawyers, and creating complicated structures intended to comply with or sidestep the statutes.

Reflections

The government's efforts to minimize fraud, kickbacks and conflicts of interest in the delivery of health care services are a case study of how the law may not always be an effective substitute for the previously presumed ethical conduct of physicians and other health care professionals. The multitude of statutes and regulations were created in response to actual and perceived abuses in the financing and delivery of health care services. The transactional philosophy of the law, wherein compliance is rewarded and non-compliance is punished, supplanted the transformational philosophy of professional ethics which should readily recognize, avoid or correct any conduct or relationship which had even the appearance of a conflict of interest and/or was not in the best interest of the patient. After more than ten years of crafting, redrafting and interpreting its laws and regulations, the government itself has challenged health care providers to not merely comply with the requirements of the law but to exceed the expectations of patients and to embrace the traditional ethical standards which should preclude the need for volumes of case law, statutes and regulations.

Lying for Patients

Despite the somewhat suffocating multitude of laws and regulations and notwithstanding the health care professional's commitment to ethical conduct, evidence has emerged to suggest that many physicians will lie to third party payers in order to protect, preserve and enhance the health and well being of their patients.

A study, first reported in the October 25, 1999 edition of the "Archives of Internal Medicine" revealed that many physicians were willing to deceive the third party payer in order to protect their patient.

105

This phenomenon is not surprising inasmuch as the "deception" engaged in is motivated not by economic self interest but by the physicians' commitment to provide medically indicated treatment which might otherwise be denied or not reimbursed. Many physicians apparently perceive their role as a patient advocate to supercede their legal obligation to obey the "law" or comply with the "ethics" of cost control.

The study indicated that doctors were more willing to mislead the payer in cases of clinical severity, e.g. coronary bypass surgery, than they were for treatments such as cosmetic rhinoplasty. The survey also indicated that physicians in markets with high managed care penetration were more likely to engage in "patient centered deception" than were those in low managed care markets.

The physicians who are willing to partake of this practice certainly violate the objective standards of both common law and statutory fraud. In an analysis utilizing the common law formula, the doctors apparently view the detriment and potential damage to their patient as a matter of greater ethical concern than any damage or detriment suffered by the system when it pays under "false pretenses" for what is medically required. Similarly, how "false" is a claim when the payment of same may mean the difference between sickness and health or even life and death? The "rationalization" of deception is justified as much as exceeding the speed limit would be justified when transporting an injured person to a hospital. Yes, the law is broken but it is violated for a "greater good".

This brief presentation is not intended to be a forum for a debate of the ethics of deceptive and illegal practices. One must, however, recognize that even laws and regulations intended to ensure truth and fairness in the marketplace of medicine may sometimes obstruct a greater truth and a more fundamental fairness of professional integrity and patient well being.

The Application of Anti-trust Laws to the Health Care "Industry"

Background

It is somewhat ironic that antitrust law has emerged as an area of concern for health care providers inasmuch as the popular perception of antitrust matters relates primarily to passing references in high school social studies class to the break up of monopolies in manufacturing and the railroad industries in the late 19th and early 20th centuries. Even the contemporary battle between the Justice Department and Microsoft seems, at first blush, alien to the administration of health care organizations. Radical changes in the delivery of health care have, however, drawn this new "industry" into the sights of the "trustbusters".

Critical Concepts

The Sherman Antitrust Act of 1890, and its evolutionary interpretation by the courts through the intervening decades, has established certain factors considered essential to establishing an antitrust violation. The elements are as follows:

1. There must exist evidence of a contract, combination or conspiracy by two or more independent parties. This requirement presumptively excludes officers, departments or divisions of the same corporation or organization.

2. The contract, combination or conspiracy must have an impact upon interstate commerce. The technological revolution and our borderless economy render virtually every business transaction one which impacts on interstate commerce.

3. The contract, combination or conspiracy must create a restraint upon trade. This restraint may be determined by one of two rules:
   A) The *per se* rule which includes conduct such as price fixing, allocations or boycotts; or
   B) The "rule of reason" wherein the court will determine not whether a particular act or practice is "reasonable" but whether it is reasonable to determine that the act or practice will be likely to have an adverse impact upon free trade.

If a plaintiff or prosecutor is able to establish the enumerated elements, the court will likely find there to be a violation of the Sherman Act.

When applying the provisions of the Sherman Act to health care cases, the courts have determined that *per se* violations are actionable. Some latitude has, however, been extended to the medical profession inasmuch as the courts will consider issues such as public service and the ethical norms of the profession when applying the "rule of reason."

The Courts have also created a "patient care defense" to antitrust charges if the accused can pass a four-part test:
   1. Was there a genuine concern for the "scientific method" in the care of the patient?;

107

2. Was the application of the "scientific method" objectively reasonable?;

3. Was the action motivated by the "scientific method" rather than economic concerns?; and

4. Could the concern for the "scientific method" been satisfied in a manner less restrictive of competition?

Few health care defendants would be able to prevail notwithstanding this special exception for health care providers.

Monopolies, Mergers and Acquisitions

The Sherman Act also prohibits monopolies by an organization if that organization: a) possesses monopoly power in a relevant market; and b) *willfully* acquires or maintains that monopoly power. Monopolies are discouraged by the law if only because they deprive consumers of meaningful choice in the marketplace. Monopoly power will be tolerated, however, if that power is attained as a result of superior product, business expertise, historical accident, patents or, in the case of health care organizations, certificates of need.

The Clayton Act regulates mergers and acquisitions if those mergers and acquisitions will tend to lessen competition and create a monopoly in a particular product line or geographic market.

Antitrust Enforcement and Health Care Organizations

The Department of Justice and the Federal Trade Commission have recognized the unique character of health care organization in terms of both their structure and the delivery of their product or service. Accordingly, the agencies have created both a "safe harbor" for small hospitals and special "Horizontal Merger Guidelines" for larger health care institutions.

The federal government will employ a five-step analysis in order to evaluate the horizontal merger of entities at the same level of production or distribution or in the same geographic market. The analysis is as follows:

1. The geographic market served by the organizations proposing a merger will be analyzed. That analysis will include an evaluation of the specific products and services offered in that geographic market.

2. The impact of any merger upon the third party payers will be assessed;

108

3.   Questions will be posed regarding the ability of new competitors to enter the market if a merger were approved;

4.   The regulators will also analyze the economic efficiencies created or likely to occur as the result of a merger or acquisition;

5.   Finally, if either party to a proposed merger or acquisition is deemed to be "failing", the merger is more likely to be approved since the preservation of competition concerns of the law would be rendered moot as a result of such a failure.

The law creates a "safe harbor" for small hospital mergers if one of the two institutions has fewer than 100 beds and has had a daily census of less than 40 patients during the three years prior to the time of the merger proposal. This exception has been created in recognition of the limited impact which a merger will have on the competitive climate of a particular market.

Pennsylvania Procedures

Pennsylvania is the only state in the Union without a state antitrust law. Absent such a statute, the Pennsylvania Office of Attorney General relies heavily upon the federal laws and guidelines noted above. In Pennsylvania, for example, the relevant geographic market for an urban hospital is considered to be a 15-mile radius while a rural hospital will enjoy a 30-mile market radius.

The Pennsylvania standards will seek to avoid market concentration but will recognize unique geographic and demographic realities as when hospital mergers were approved in both Williamsport and Hazleton. In effect, those markets were deemed to be one-hospital communities with more than one hospital.

The organizational status of the hospital, for profit vs. not for profit, will also be a significant factor to be considered in any merger or acquisition application. In the case of a not-for-profit hospital converting to or being acquired by a for profit entity, the fair market value of the former's assets must be established and the monetary value of those assets paid to a replacement not-for-profit entity. In effect, the tax and charitable benefits enjoyed by a non-profit health care organization cannot become a windfall for an acquiring or new for-profit corporation.

Reflections

Although virtually every commercial corporation and every for profit or non-profit health care organization publicly espouses a "mission statement" of some sort, the unique and inspiring missions and visions of so many health care organizations have been blurred by the passage of time and the harsh realities of contemporary market forces. Whether it be the legacy of Moses Taylor to provide health care for coal miners and their families; the religious mission of the Sisters of Mercy to minister to the temporal and spiritual needs of an immigrant population; or the mission of Robert Packer to care for the geographically isolated railroad workers, those mandates and missions cannot and should not be subsumed by mergers and acquisitions which create monopolies manipulated by the "bottom line".

Conclusion

Laws enacted to combat fraud and prevent unfair market dominance are clearly intended to protect and enhance the "common good". Unfortunately, we have become a litigious society so dominated by lawyers that the simple principles of truth and justice have become obscured by the "new" American way. The joke that two lawyers in a room will produce three opinions, combined with the fact that there are more lawyers practicing in Washington D.C. than in all of Japan, should give us cause for concern. Our laws may serve as both a sword and a shield but they will never supplant and can only supplement a personal and organizational commitment to "do the right thing".

(Some material for this presentation was referenced from "Healthcare Law and Ethics: Issues for the Age of Managed Care", by Dean M. Harris, Health Administration Press, Chicago, Illinois (1999))

NOTES:

NOTES:

112

Chapter 6

Health Economics and Managed Care
Economics for Directors in Managed Care Era

Fevzi Akinci, Ph.D.

The health care system in the United States is evolving at an unprecedented rate. Consumer demands for a greater choice of health plans and providers, purchaser drives to control rising health care costs, changing population demographics, and development of new and often expensive technologies for managing care have stimulated significant changes in the health care market over the past several years. The growth of managed care has been explosive in both private and public sectors in the past decade, fundamentally changing the way health care services are provided and delivered to the ultimate consumers. Managed care is now the dominant form of coverage for privately insured individuals. Approximately 80 million U.S. citizens are enrolled in Health Maintenance Organizations (HMOs), roughly 29.2 percent of the U.S. population (Coile, 2000). Medicaid managed care enrollment exceeded 55 percent in 2000. While enrollment in Medicare managed care lags behind, with approximately 17 percent beneficiaries receiving their services from some type of managed care program, there is a greater growth potential for this program given the provisions of the 1997 Balanced Budget Act to expand Medicare+Choice (HCFA, 2001). While managed care has become the mainstream delivery system for health services for many, it has challenged policymakers, purchasers, health care managers, and consumers since its creation.

A solid understanding of the forces that have given rise to managed care, common organizational models of it, and financial incentives created by managed care is essential for health care managers and directors to successfully lunch effective strategies in this rapidly changing environment. To that end, this chapter first examines the forces in U.S. health care system that have given rise to managed care and discusses the current managed care structures in marketplace. Key economic theories of the firm are presented next to help you understand the economic behaviors of health care providers in the new era of managed care. Finally, a review of financial incentives under alternative payment arrangements is offered to inform you about the challenges and opportunities associated with each payment system as well as the appropriate steps that need to be taken to assure future financial viability of your organizations.

113

Health Care System Change and Emergence of Managed Care

In 1999, Americans spent 1.2 trillion on health care representing 13 percent of gross domestic product (GDP) (HCFA, 2001). GDP measures total current domestic expenditures for goods and services by consumers, business, and government. The national health care spending as a percentage of total spending was only 5.7 percent in 1965 (Campbell, et al 1998). While the United States continues to spend considerably more per capita on health care ($4,178 in 1998) than any other developed country, it compares poorly on a number of available outcome indicators. Indicators for which the United States showed the greatest relative decline since 1960 include life expectancy at birth for females, life expectancy at age sixty for females, and infant mortality (Anderson and Hussey, 2001). These results suggest that more spending does not always produce better health.

Health insurance continues to be expensive with premium increases exceeding 8 percent in 2000 after remaining under 4 percent from 1995 through 1998. Premium increases are expected to be even higher in 2001 (Gabel, 2000). Today, there are approximately 43 million uninsured people, nearly 10 million more than a decade ago (Ginsburg, 2001). With expected health insurance premium increases in the near future, the numbers of uninsured and underinsured are likely to be even higher. As the economy falters and labor markets loosen, employers are already reducing health benefits and shifting more cost to employees. The rising number of uninsured is also expected to increase the burden on our nation's safety net providers. Indeed inner-city hospitals, community health centers and other safety net providers are already facing financial pressures from managed care and cuts in federal subsidies.

Before 1965, the federal government assumed rather limited responsibility for financing health care services in the United States. Only workers and their families received tax-subsidized health insurance coverage for major medical expenses through their employers. Many policies were implemented in the 1950s and 1960s to increase access to health care services culminating in Medicare and Medicaid legislation in 1965. This legislation provided health insurance coverage to the elderly through Medicare and to the poor through Medicaid programs. During the 1970s, health care expenditures and health insurance premiums rose significantly and health care reform efforts turned from expanding access to containing expenditures. With the failure of serious health reform efforts at the federal level, managed care has emerged as the primary market reform attempt to contain health care costs in a system that is widely believed to be highly inefficient.

114

According to Lee (2000) there are three basic problems with traditional open-ended fee-for-service plans. First, they encourage the use of covered services by consumers and providers as long as the direct cost to consumers is less than the direct benefit. Second, they discourage use of uncovered services by consumers, even highly effective ones. And finally, the prices paid by consumers and the prices received by providers do not reflect either provider costs or consumer valuations. Obviously there is limited incentive under such a payment system to promote efficient use of resources or to improve the health of a defined population.

However, one should remember that such goals were not a major focus of attention in health policy during the mid and well into the late 20th century. Today, managed care is changing the incentives created by these open ended fee-for-service plans by using a number of directed organizational structures and techniques. Some examples of these include the use of gate keeping with prior authorizations for hospital services and referrals, utilization review programs, and global or partial capitation payments for providers.

Managed Care Defined

What is managed care? Indeed, it is not easy to define managed care given its continuous modification and varying perceptions by key players in the health care market place. Proponents define managed care as a continuum of arrangements designed to organize, finance, and deliver health care services in the most effective and efficient manner to a defined population. Williams and Torrens (1999) define manage care as "an organized effort by health insurance plans and providers to use financial incentives and organizational arrangements to alter provider and patient behavior so that health care services are delivered and utilized in a more efficient and lower-cost manner" (p. 152). Under managed care, the financing and delivery of health care are organized by a single entity. Whatever the exact definition, managed care clearly dominates the current health care market. According to the American Association of Health Plans (AAHP), managed care organizations (MCOs) are entities that offer an HMO, preferred provider organization (PPO), or point of service (POS) plan, or any combination of these (AAHP, 1997). The following section briefly describes different models of managed care organizations and current trends in health plan enrollment.

Managed Care Models and Current Trends

HMOs are managed care organizations that provide a comprehensive set of health care services to a defined population for a fixed monthly fee by contracting with or employing physicians, hospitals, and other health care providers. Staff model HMOs directly employ salaried physicians, whereas group model HMOs contract with a limited number of group practices. The typical payment system for physicians in group model HMOs is capitation (per member, per month-PMPM) with incentives. The most common models of HMOs are Independent Practice Association (IPAs) and network models. The IPAs contract with both large and small groups of physicians, and even with solo practice physicians, to provide care to HMO members in the physicians' own offices. An HMO that uses several contracting methods is often called a network-model HMO and contracts with several large multispecialty groups or IPAs. Another common form of managed care organization is a Preferred Provider Organization (PPO). PPOs can be defined as networks of hospitals, physicians, and other health care providers that provide medical care to individuals for a negotiated fee. Unlike HMOs, PPOs do not assume financial risk of arranging for health care benefits. Finally, Point of Service (POS) plans resemble a combination of a PPO and an IPA, allowing access to out-of-network providers for a higher copay by patients and paying some providers through methods other than discounted fee-for-service.

Early examples of managed care arrangements were typically characterized by the voluntary participation of employees, workers, and physicians. In most cases, employers created prepaid health care arrangements in order to attract and retain their workers. The participation of physicians in early forms of prepaid medical care, however, was difficult to achieve given that many of those who chose to participate risked expulsion from local medical societies and license revocation. The Western Clinic in Tacoma, Washington, is sometimes cited as the first example of an HMO, or prepaid group practice as it was known until the early 1970s. The federal HMO Act of 1973 fostered the development of HMOs across the country. This was accomplished through a combination of awarding sizable federal grants and loans for the creation HMOs, superseding state laws restricting the formation of HMOs, requiring employers to offer federally-qualified HMOs, and establishing a voluntary qualification process for HMOs (Knight, 1998).

Traditional indemnity health insurance through comprehensive coverage of hospital services and small co-payments for medical services, lessened patient concerns with hospital and medical expenses. Physicians were reimbursed largely on a fee-for-service basis with limited financial responsibility for hospital inpatient use. Hospitals encouraged increased utilization of their services by providing incentives to loyal physicians and physician groups. There was also a rapid introduction of new medical technologies, often actively encouraged through financial incentives by

116

providers, without adequate concern regarding effectiveness. This was encouraged because of the generous insurer reimbursement policies for use and purchase costs. The overall intent of managed care, therefore, was to eliminate unnecessary and inappropriate services and use less costly institutional settings without reducing quality. First generation managed care plans used restrictive techniques, such as selective contracting, gate keeping, and stringent utilization review programs to control the use of health care services by both providers and consumers. Initial managed care savings were largely attributable to lower utilization of hospital services and deep provider price discounts. Some of these savings were offset by burgeoning administrative costs. Given the excess capacity among hospitals and physicians, HMOs were successful in shifting large numbers of their enrollees to providers who competed almost exclusively on cost to be included in the HMO provider network. In the 1980s and 1990s, for-profit HMOs competing with fee-for-service plans enjoyed double-digit growth in profit margins (Williams and Torrens, 1999).

In order to achieve further reductions in medical costs, so called second-generation managed care approaches relied more on changing providers' practice patterns, decreasing inappropriate use of services, and substituting less costly in-home services for lengthy stays in the hospital. As the managed care plans began to shift more of the capitation risk to physicians and hospitals, providers were given financial incentives to develop new approaches for delivering medical care services with a greater emphasis being placed on improving individual patient outcomes and enhancing the health status of defined populations (Feldstein, 1999). Under a capitated payment arrangement, providers have the potential to enjoy the benefits of treatment innovation and cost-reduction efforts. Providers have come to understand that there are also risks involved in these arrangements.

One of the most important changes in the U.S. health care system over the past several years has been the development of a virulent backlash against managed care. Backed by consumers' demand for a grater choice of plans and providers, physicians' dissatisfaction with the loss of autonomy and reduced fees, and purchasers' desire for greater accountability and value for dollars spent, the backlash against managed care has intensified in recent years and has begun to have visible effects on local markets (Lesser and Ginsburg, 2000). Managed care's retreat is predicted to lead to higher costs, more cost sharing for consumers, new barriers to access, greater numbers of uninsured, and a weaker platform from which to improve quality of care (Ginsburg, 2001).

Today, HMO growth has slowed as the managed care market has become saturated. Since consumers like freedom of choice, flexibility, and cost control offered by loosely structured models of managed care, many traditional HMOs are losing market share. Slower-than-expected growth in HMO enrollment was reported in all twelve randomly selected markets representative of metropolitan areas by a recent Center for Studying Health System Change research (Lesser and Ginsburg, 2000). Despite earlier predictions, enrollees in preferred provider organizations (PPOs) were found to be less likely to switch to HMO products. In fact, a rapid growth in PPO enrollment was noted in many markets. Broad and inclusive provider networks are becoming the norm in many markets across the nation. Especially POS and "open access" products are gaining more share of these markets with their out-of-network coverage and direct access to certain specialty providers.

On the supply side of the health care market, many providers and health plans are abandoning their vertical integration strategies that were once envisioned as the future of health care. Significant investment of energy and capital as well as cultural differences between health plan and provider staffs are often cited as the main obstacles to vertical integration efforts (Lesser and Ginsburg, 2000). Today, increased emphasis on horizontal consolidation and active pursuit of broad geographic scope constitute the prevailing strategies of many provider organizations. Most of the hospital merger activity that sought to enhance the hospital's indispensability to health plan networks and achieve economies of scale in response to the competitive threats has now slowed down. However, Lesser and Ginsberg (2000) note that despite increased concentration of ownership, there has been limited consolidation of services or capacity. They argue that the desire of institutions to maintain a full spectrum of services across a broad geographic area and thereby attract managed care contracts and increase referral bases has worked against the closing of underutilized duplicative services in neighboring markets and even creates incentives to expand services and excess capacity in many communities. While mergers have helped hospitals to increase their market power, efficiency gains have been limited by a number of factors. As mentioned earlier, in many cases hospitals have been reluctant to make significant changes in the organization of their care delivery systems. Consolidation of clinical services and capacity would yield more significant efficiency gains than integrating so called "back-room" functions such as purchasing and finance (Lesser and Brewster, 2001).

Some analysts view the movement away from integrated delivery systems and capitated payment of providers as key aspects of the retreat from

118

managed care. This retreat may remove a potential platform for providers to improve quality since such systems have in theory the potential to improve quality through the use of evidence-based medicine applied to the needs of a defined population (Ginsburg, 2001). In practice there is little evidence to suggest that these systems actually do improve population health. Finally, increasing network instability is creating additional access barriers in a number of communities. Many providers are declining to renew their contracts with managed care plans largely due to disagreements over payment rates. This not only disrupts the continuum of care for consumers but also forces them to pay more out-of-pocket expenses (Short et al, 2001).

A close examination of key "economic theories of the firm" would be helpful for directors not only to better understand the economic behavior of hospitals in the evolving managed care environment but also to devise effective business strategies for success.

Economic Theory of the Firm

The theory of the firm states that firms are willing and able to enter a competitive market to produce goods or to supply services under certain conditions (Pindyck & Rubinfeld, 1989). A firm will continue to supply the quantity of goods and services demanded by consumers as long as the revenues it receives exceed the expenses incurred during production; that is, the firm's economic incentive to enter or leave the market is based on the ability to make a profit. The theory further states that in a competitive market, an organization will institute processes that promote operational efficiencies, which, in turn, contribute to the ability to remain competitive and profitable within that market.

While the classical economics view of firms in competitive markets is that they seek to minimize costs and maximize profits (Pindyck & Rubinfeld, 1989), it is important to note an alternate theory. The central proposition of the X-efficiency theory states that "not all firms minimize costs; that is, not all firms produce on the outer bounds of their production possibility surfaces" (DeAlessie, 1983). This is the case because assumptions of a perfectly competitive market do not hold for some markets, and in health care in particular there are wide variations from perfect competition. Using the individual as a unit of analysis, this theory emphasizes the role of behavioral/motivational variables inside the firm in order to explain the reasons for departures from cost minimizing behavior. In addition, several external variables, such as degree of market competition, size of the firm, type of ownership, and regulatory environment are also identified within the

X-efficiency framework that might result in little managerial effort for cost minimization (Frantz, 1985; Rosko, Chilingerian, Zinn, & Aaronson, 1995).

Other Economic Theories

According to economic theory, services in the public or not-for-profit sector are likely to be produced less efficiently than in the private sector. This is explained mainly by the lack of profit motive in the public or not-for-profit sector (Goldman & Grossman, 1983). Much of the research effort in health services literature has, therefore, focused on the impact of ownership type on efficiency of health care organizations. While a large number of studies have found that for-profit health care organizations are more efficient than their not-for-profit counterparts, some studies do not report any significant differences in the efficiency between the two types of organizations (Rosko, et al., 1995).

According to property rights theory of the firm, different structures of property rights conveyed by different institutional arrangements can affect the efficiency of firms (Fizel & Nunnikhoven, 1992). More specifically, owners of proprietary firms have exclusive rights to retain (or distribute) the equity or residual value that is in excess of the financial obligations the firms have incurred during their operation (Frech, 1976), with the resulting incentive to closely monitor inputs, and productivity and to produce efficiently (Fizel & Nunnikhoven, 1992). On the other hand, in the case of not-for-profit firms, the owners' property rights to income are attenuated and non-pecuniary goods are consumed at the expense of efficiency and wealth creation (Fizel & Nunnikhoven, 1992). Because profits accrue to owners of for-profit firms, they have a reason to minimize costs and are more likely to strive for efficiency. Owners of non-profit firms are generally assumed to maximize size, quality, and slack, each of which may contribute to inefficiency (Fizel & Nunnikhoven, 1993). Similarly, the public choice literature suggests that decision makers in hierarchical, not-for-profit institutions are more likely to pursue budget-maximization behaviors rather than cost-minimization behaviors (Niskanen, 1968).

Both property rights and public choice theories further maintain that incentives to maximize profits in not-for-profit organizations are attenuated because these firms serve multiple constituents and have multiple goals. Some of the goals of health care organizations, such as serving as a safety net for the uninsured and providing employment opportunities for local citizens, may not be consistent with minimizing total costs and maximizing profits. In addition, the presence of federal subsidies (Rosko, et al., 1995) and cost-

120

based reimbursement (Goldman & Grossman, 1983) may promote inefficiencies in the production of health care services.

Tuckman and Chang (1988) argued, however, that the effect of ownership status on efficiency can be less significant if one accounts for the competitive factors that prevail in a market. Referring specifically to the nursing home industry, the authors claimed that when competition in a market is substantial, institutional survival requires cost minimization for homes of all ownership types.

The X-efficiency theory developed by Liebenstein (1980) similarly suggests that the behavior and cost structures of not-for-profit firms will converge with those of for-profit firms when environmental pressures threaten their survival (Rosko, et al., 1995). This prediction is especially relevant in today's increasingly competitive health care delivery system as managed care arrangements are rapidly replacing the heretofore-standard fee-for-service payment system for many health care providers.

Nature of Financial Incentives Under Alternative Payment Arrangements

One of the fundamental changes that has taken place in the U.S. health care system over the past decade is the shift away from fee-for-service payment mechanisms to capitated and other incentive-payment system arrangements, particularly in the private health insurance market (Etheredge, 1996; Rice, 1997). The shift from the cost-plus environment of the 1960s and 1970s to the fixed-fee environment of the 1980s and 1990s has forced health care managers and directors to pay more close attention to operational efficiency (Feldstein, 1985-86; Kleinsorge & Karney, 1992). In addition, over the past two decades, the economic risk for providing health care services has been systematically shifted from the insurers to the providers.

A clear understanding of the concept of economic risk is essential to fully comprehend and differentiate between the incentive structures of cost-based or fee-for-service and capitated payment systems. According to Campbell, Schmitz, & Waller (1998), the two components of economic risk for providing health care to a defined population are: "… the price risk and the risk associated with the volume of services used. In turn, the volume risk is made up of two parts: the actuarial risk of illness in the population that is being covered and the risk of over using resources. Thus, the costs to a risk taker to provide health services to a defined population will be a combination of the price that is charged for those services and the volume of services used. To the extent that either or both of these two variables can be

121

rationally controlled, the risk taker stands a better chance of being successful and making a profit" (p. 75).

Although there has been a great deal of research conducted on the impact of capitation versus fee-for-service payment systems on behaviors of health care providers (with more of the research focusing on physician behavior), little has been conducted on different incentives within managed care plans (Rice, 1997). In general, the existing literature provides strong evidence of lower service utilization and expenditures by managed care enrollees than by persons with conventional fee-for-service coverage. This is achieved without any apparent adverse impact on quality of care of studied populations (Miller & Luft, 1997).

One of the key concerns with capitated payment arrangements is the likelihood of under provision of necessary services by health care providers to patients (Blumenthal, 1996; Williams & Torrens, 1999). Proponents of capitation argue that the financial incentive to under use services is no more a conflict than the incentive to overuse in the fee-for-service payment system. Opponents, on the other hand, maintain that it is fundamentally unethical for physicians to be paid more to do less (Reagan, 1987; Watchel & Stein, 1993). Unfortunately, little empirical data is available to determine whether or not capitation actually results in under provision of necessary medical services (Williams & Torrens, 1999).

Financial incentive systems in managed care plans for physicians generally consist of two parts. The first part consists of basic compensation arrangements including salary, fee-for-service, and capitation. The second part consists of incentive schemes to influence the use of hospital or specialist services (Kwon, 1996). Some examples of so called "mixed model" or "partial capitation" methods include the following arrangements (Rice, 1997): First is the withholding of some percentage of payment due to physicians, and not returning it if the physician hospitalizes or refers patients to specialists more often than considered appropriate. Such withholds can be based on an individual physician's performance, or on the performance of the physician group as a whole. Second is subjecting the physician to financial risks over and above the withhold amounts. Third is providing bonus payments to physicians if at the end of a financial period there exists a surplus in hospitalization or specialty referral risk pools. Again, these bonuses can be determined based on either the individual physician's performance or the performance of a group of physicians as a whole. The risk pools that are based on the performance of a group of physicians, however, may not be as effective as those based on the individual physician's performance in terms of the desired behavior change because of the potential

122

problem of "free-riding". A final arrangement consists of placing the physician at financial risk for tests or other procedures that they order.

According to Gold and others (1995), fifty-seven percent of network and independent practice association (IPA) HMOs reported having capitation arrangements with their primary care physicians, and approximately 80 percent also withheld funds (or offered bonuses) as an incentive to limit referrals in 1994. The three U.S. studies reviewed by Rice (1997) to determine the impact of capitation on physician behavior in HMOs indicated a trend towards more conservative use of resources by physicians who were reimbursed based on capitation and the other incentive mechanisms described above.

In the first study, which examined the impact of various physician compensation methods in HMOs on service utilization, it was found that compared to fee-for-service, salaried physicians had 13 percent lower hospitalization rates while capitation lowered these rates by 8 percent. This study also indicated that putting individual physicians at risk for deficits in referral funds, and having the level of risk exceed the amount of withhold, reduced visits per enrollee by approximately 10 percent (Hillman, Pauly, & Kerstein, 1989).

The second study was based on a single HMO (IPA model) in Wisconsin, which changed its payment system to its primary care physicians from fee-for-service to capitation, with risk sharing for hospital and specialists services in 1983. The results of this study indicated that one year later primary care visits increased 18 percent, while referrals to specialists outside the group declined by 45 percent. In addition, hospital admissions and lengths of stay were reported to have declined by 16.3 percent and 12 percent respectively in the second year of implemented changes in reimbursement (Stearns, Wolfe, & Kindig, 1992).

Similar to the second study, the final study reviewed by Rice (1997) examined the impact of a change in payment from fee-for-service with a 15 percent withhold to capitation for primary care physicians in Illinois. Capitation payment also included shared risk for specialist services and a bonus if hospitalization rates were held below a threshold level. This study found that specialist costs increased 2 percent after the payment method change, after increasing 12 percent in previous years. It was also noted that the cost of hospital outpatient services declined 7 percent, after increasing 12 percent in previous years. However, no effect was detected on hospital utilization in this study (Ogden, Carlson, & Bernstein, 1990).

Two more recent studies examining the impact of managed care on provider behavior (one on physician and another on hospitals) are summarized here. Burns, Chilingerian and Wholey (1994) explored variations in the use of hospital resources across individual physicians using hospital discharge data over a two-year period (1989-1990) for 43,625 women undergoing Cesarean sections and vaginal deliveries without complications. Researchers defined the efficiency of physician practices as "the degree of variation in patient charges and length of stay below the average of treating all patients with the same condition in the same hospital in the same year with the same severity of illness, controlling for discharge status and the presence of complications" (Burns, Chilingerian, and Wholey, 1994, p.583). It was found that in addition to individual physician characteristics (years of experience, board certification, and graduation from a foreign medical school), efficiency was influenced by practice organization factors such as patient volume and managed care load. Specifically, the statistical analysis indicated that physicians with larger practices and a higher share of managed care patients seem to be more efficient. However, the effect of managed care on efficiency was statistically significant only for vaginal delivery patients.

Conrad et al. (1996) studied the impact of individual dimensions of hospital managed care strategies on hospital efficiency using cost per discharge as the dependent variable. The authors examined 21,135 inpatient discharges in 1991 and 23,262 discharges in 1992 performed by thirty-seven member hospitals of seven health systems in the Pacific, Rocky Mountain, and Southwest regions of the United States. Of the three dimensions of hospital managed care strategy studied, the one that was shown to be consistently related to lower cost per discharge was the proportion of hospital revenues derived from per case or capitation payment. The statistical analysis showed that hospitals with a higher percentage of revenues from managed care contracts paying on a capitation or per case basis had significantly lower cost per discharge, controlling for other variables in the regression analysis. The other two dimensions that were also found to be related to the efficiency of inpatient resource use included the hospital's mechanism for sharing information on resource consumption with clinicians and the use of formalized, systematic care coordination mechanisms.

Given the evidence from other providers, it is likely that the evolving managed care environment is also forcing hospitals to think more competitively and to operate more efficiently in order to survive. Before 1983, hospitals have relied on the traditional cost-based payment system. Medicare and Medicaid have traditionally reimbursed hospitals based on the allowable cost of providing the services. In this setting, the economic risk for providing health care services to hospital patients rests with the payer.

Practically speaking, there is no way for a hospital to lose money on these patients under this reimbursement system. As a hospital provides more patient services or procedures, it receives more reimbursement, and as a result, cost-based reimbursement provides limited, if any, incentives for operational efficiency and cost control for hospitals. In fact, Campbell, et al. (1998) argued that "A 100 percent cost-based provider would not be financially motivated to achieve an efficient use of resources" (p. 129).

Since the early 1980s, both the government and the private sector have been demanding greater efficiency of the health care delivery system. Cost-based reimbursement for hospitals under Medicare has given way to payment based on fixed prices (Diagnostic Related Groups-DRGs) under Prospective Payment System (PPS) system. This new payment reform requires that reimbursement for hospital services be on the basis of predetermined fee for each diagnosis. Price competition among hospitals and physicians increased after this policy change in reimbursement as insurance companies, in turn, compete on the basis of premiums in the sale of group health insurance. With the PPS, the payer shifted an additional volume risk to the provider by making the provider primarily responsible for the length of stay of the patient. In other words, the provider assumes risk associated with the price, the consumption of resources, and the length of stay. The only risk that remains with the payer is the risk for frequency of illness in the population.

The capitation payment system represents the final step in the shifting of economic risk from insurers to providers (Campbell, et al., 1998). Capitation refers to reimbursing the hospital on a per member per month basis to cover all institutional costs for a defined population of members. The payment varies by age and gender but does not fluctuate with premium revenue. It is very important for a hospital to know what exactly is covered under the capitation payment, what is not covered, and to perform aggressive utilization management to assure appropriate use of medical services. The capitated hospital also needs to have stop-loss insurance to protect it against catastrophic cases (Kongstvedt, 2001). It is important, however, to note the various models of capitation that can be found in practice. As indicated earlier, examples of these include global capitation; capitation with additional financial risk, with withholds and/or bonuses; and with carve-outs based on type of service (e.g., preventive care), diagnoses and conditions (e.g., AIDS), and referral specialty (e.g., ophthalmology) (Bodenheimer & Grumbach, 1996).

Under a global capitated payment system, a health provider receives a fixed fee per member per month (PMPM) in return for guaranteed provision of a pre-defined range of health services (Rice, 1997). If a health provider can provide the services for less than the capitation payment, it keeps the difference. If the provider's costs exceed the capitation revenue, it absorbs the excess costs. Under a cost-based arrangement, a health provider receives more reimbursement each time it serves a patient; however with a capitation payment arrangement, each time a prepaid patient service is provided it represents a reduction from the per member per month premium already received. Therefore, Campbell, et al. (1998) maintain that "... unlike cost-based reimbursement that encourages a health care organization to increase reimbursable costs, capitation rewards less costly and more efficient approaches to treatment" (p.146).

It is important to note that unlike under the cost-based reimbursement system, survival under the capitated payment system is directly related to the health care provider's ability to manage its costs. Under a fully capitated payment arrangement, the payer shifts all the economic risk to the provider including the price, the risk for resource use, and the risk for illness in the population. Therefore, the health care provider now has every incentive to be more efficient in service delivery. Participation in a capitation scheme will require that hospitals rethink their approach to staffing and equipment to ensure the most efficient and appropriate mix and number of scarce resources. They must also pay close attention to patients' length of stay, ensuring that each patient remains hospitalized only as long as medically necessary, and use referrals to specialists more judiciously in order to remain financially solvent.

What determines the advantage and disadvantage of each method is the rate of reimbursement. As long as the rate of reimbursement is high enough to cover total costs, inefficient hospitals will survive in a cost-based or fee-for service reimbursement environment. However, under the managed care scenario, the determination of efficiency depends heavily on the performance of the most efficient or best practice hospitals included in the area. In a market characterized by increased competition, the most efficient hospital will survive and prosper while others will either fail or be forced to become more efficient.

To summarize, if health care providers do not have appropriate incentives to be efficient, it is difficult to achieve economic efficiency in the provision of medical services. Health care providers confront mixed incentives for both inefficient and efficient production in today's health care market. Under the traditional cost-based system, the overall incentive is to "do more," because more services lead to increased revenues. With its greater emphasis on resource consumption and efficiency, the capitated reimbursement system contradicts the traditional "more-is-better" approach to health care (Hillman,

1991). Under capitation, there are strong financial incentives to "do less" by providing fewer services and minimizing costs (Hellinger, 1996).

Discussion and Conclusion

Faced with increased pressure from managed care organizations and other health care purchasers, hospitals have moved rapidly in the 1990s to gain greater control over the appropriateness and cost effectiveness, as well as quality, of the care provided. The shift in reimbursement toward prospective payment have significantly changed the financial incentives for hospitals, requiring them to ensure that hospital admissions are justifiable, that lengths of stay do not exceed accepted norms, and that treatment regimens are medically appropriate. Evidence-based practice guidelines, continuous quality improvement techniques, and withholding and risk sharing arrangement have become commonplace with hospital medical staffs, particularly under health plan contracts with fixed payments. The growing pressure on hospitals to exercise greater influence over physician behavior to contain costs and control utilization and improve quality and outcomes is indeed a significant threat to physician autonomy and may contribute to greater conflict between hospitals and physicians over what has become a shrinking pie of opportunity for reimbursement. Some of the common methods used by hospitals to influence physician behavior have included direct appeals, joint ventures between medical services and technology, economic credentialing, employment of physicians (Glandon and Morrisey, 1986), education, peer review and feedback, administrative rules, participation in developing treatment guidelines, and incentives (Grieco and Eisenberg, 1993).

In those markets that are heavily penetrated by managed care, hospitals and physicians have pursued a number of strategies varying in response to the leverage that managed care plans had in the selection of providers and the pricing of managed care products.   Integrated physician/hospital organizations (PHO) have been formed in certain markets to share the risk and benefits of managed care contracting. On the other hand, intense competition for ambulatory care services and health plan contracts has left hospitals struggling to utilize excess capacity as their physicians migrate to other facilities, or consider selling their assets to practice management companies (Williams and Torrens, 1999). In recent years, however, many of these so called provider intermediary organizations appear to have stumbled badly. Unrealistic expectations concerning risk contracting is often cited to be a key factor in the failures of these organizations. For example, PHOs, commonly led and controlled by hospital administrators, often could not garner the trust of physicians. Physicians often found that PHOs negotiate

127

contracts with plans that are good deals for the hospital but not for the participating physicians. The health plans also seem to be reluctant to delegate financial risk and associated responsibility for care management to a PHO that could potentially exert significant market power. (Lesser and Ginsburg, 2000).

A few years ago, most observers of health system change believed that capitation would become the dominant method of payment for health care services. However, recent evidence suggest that the use of capitation to pay providers has stagnated in most markets with a number of communities seeing major disruption of services because of the failures of organizations that had accepted extensive capitated risk (Lesser and Ginsburg, 2000). Lack of administrative skills and data, not having a large enough capitated patient base, and inadequate risk adjustment are some key factors that have dampened the enthusiasm of most providers for capitation (Lee, 2000). As health plans are moving away from tightly managed care products and providers are gaining more clout, the decline in risk-based payment arrangements is likely to weaken this mechanism of cost control in the U.S. health care system. Ginsburg (2001) also notes that the absence of capitation payment undermines one aspect of the business case for providers to engage in quality improvement activities. He argues that when a hospital is paid on a per diem basis, any initiatives to reduce length of stay detract from the bottom line. Similarly, when disease management programs have significant educational components or require investment in information systems by physician practices paid under fee-for-service arrangement, the practices are not adequately compensated for these additional expenditures. Therefore, Ginsburg (2001) concludes that "The potential exists for disease management and other such programs to fall out of favor, leaving patients facing fractured, uncoordinated and, potentially, poor-quality care" (p. 7). While it is difficult to predict the compensation arrangements for providers ten years from now, it appears that a form of the fee-for-service system remains the norm for today with some hybrid payment arrangements such as withholds and utilization-adjusted fee schedules.

It is clear that today's external competitive pressures are forcing hospitals to reexamine their goals, priorities, and programs while increasing the need for clearer direction and stronger leadership by the board of directors. Boards have the often difficult task of balancing the institution's overall mission, quality, and community benefit as well as seeking to compete effectively. Pointer, Alexander and Zuckerman (1995) suggest that rather than making decisions about management actions, such as approval of construction plans, budget changes, physician privileges, and response to malpractice events, boards will be increasingly shaping and making complex strategic decisions, such as investment in recruitment of primary care physicians, clinical integration in merged or affiliated organizations, and investment in information technology and radical improvements of quality and service to customers. Therefore, board members are increasingly required to understand the long-term implications of these important business decisions. So, it is time to rise to the new challenges and become a more informed, involved, and effective leader of change in your organization.

NOTES:

Chapter 7

Finance and Accounting Issues in Health Care
Health Insurance Coverage, Retirement and the Elderly

Barry H. Williams, JD, MT, MBA, CPA
Associate Professor of Accounting
King's College, Wilkes-Barre, PA

Fevzi Akinci, Ph.D.
Assistant Professor of Health Care Administration
King's College, Wilkes-Barre, PA

Introduction

People living in the United States today can expect to live longer than their parents and grandparents. Improvements in the diagnostic and surgical procedures utilized by physicians and other medical providers, prescription drug developments and lifestyle factors have lengthened life expectancies (Jefferson 685). During the course of the 20th century, the life expectancy at birth has increased 60 percent to 76.7 years while the life expectancy at an attained age of 65 has increased from 11.9 years in 1900 to 17.8 reported for 1998, or a 50 percent increase. While the life expectancy has been rising, the death rate for the period 1980 through 1997 has declined by 16 percent for the age population between 65 and 74 and 4 percent for those 85 and older (CDC 59). This combination of trend lines would indicate a continued increase in life expectancies into the 21st century.

At the same time, as life expectancies are increasing the reported health profile of the senior population indicates a worsening health condition than those of the younger population groups (CDC 53). In 2000 the estimated population of persons age 65 and older is reported at 13 percent of the total population of the United States or an estimated 35 million persons. This population is expected to rise to an approximate 20 percent of the total population of the United States with the number of persons increasing to 70 million persons (CDC 53). Out of this estimated population of the age group 65 and older, the percent of non-institutionalized persons was 96 percent (CDC 55). When considering a reported 28 percent of non-institutionalized persons 65 years of age and older reporting their health status as fair or poor, an estimated 18.8 million persons will be reporting in this category (CDC 55). The result of an aging population with an increasing number in the declining health category would project to increasing demand for health-related services. This upward trend of the senior population, those 65 years of age and older, is estimated to cause the expenditures for health care to increase from $300 million to an estimated $750 million (CDC 69).

While the trend toward declining health through the risks of disease increases with age, a number of measures for the prevention or mitigation of this declining health trend exist. Principle amongst those measures is:

- Promoting a Healthy Lifestyle. Avoidance of unhealthy practices such as smoking and excessive use of alcohol along with regular physical activity;
- Early Detection Practices. Routinely having appropriate health screening and follow up care;
- Immunization. Reduction in the incidence of such diseases as pneumonia and influenza can result;
- Reduced injuries. Increasing regular physical activity and being aware of the physical environment in which we live (CDC 69-70).

Whether living a healthy lifestyle impacts a persons future health is relatively unpredictable, persons must prepare for the current and future medical costs related to the possibility of these health concerns. A person's financial security for daily living and retirement will be impacted negatively if health issues are not corrected. The increase in life expectancy coupled with the declining death rate has impacted government tax policy due to the potential ramifications of health care costs. The Internal Revenue Code of 1986 includes an increasing number of tax-related provisions to encourage persons to save money for retirement in anticipation of the need for financial security in the future. Tax policy which encourages retirement savings allows taxpayers to save money prior to the payment of tax on the income set aside with the additional provision that persons cannot withdraw the funds until at or near retirement age unless they pay a penalty. In addition, employers are offered tax incentives to encourage sponsoring different types of retirement programs for their employees.

When a retirement program sponsored by an employer meets the requirement set forth in the Internal Revenue Code to provide for the deferral of tax to the employee and a current tax deduction to the employer, it is considered a "qualified plan." Examples of these include:

- Individual Retirement Accounts, Regular and Roth. Contributions to a regular IRA are deductible to the taxpayer when the contribution is made with the tax on the earnings postponed until the funds are withdrawn. The purpose of this postponement of tax is to assist the taxpayer in the accumulation of retirement funds through the ability

132

to create earnings on the deferred tax liability that will accrue to the taxpayer (Internal Revenue Code §219). The Roth IRA does not permit the taxpayer to take a tax deduction at the time of contribution to the fund, the benefit accrues at the time of withdrawal when the taxpayer pays no income tax upon the withdrawals (Internal Revenue Code §408A).

- Keogh Plans. Self-employed taxpayers are permitted to set up retirement programs which provide for higher contribution limits than the IRA accounts. While presented with a benefit of greater retirement savings for the self-employed the cost to the employer is the requirement of covering employees under the plan (Internal Revenue Code §§401-404).

- Employer Pension Plans. Employers are permitted to create various types of qualified pensions plans that allow the employer and the employee to make contributions to the plan providing a tax deduction to the employer while deferring income to the employee. These plans come within two broad categories: Defined Benefit Plans and Defined Contribution Plans. Under a defined benefit plan the employee is promised a specific benefit upon retirement (Internal Revenue Code §414). Under a defined contribution plan the employee is given a specified level of contributions with the benefit fluctuating dependent upon investment performance (Internal Revenue Code §414).

While the types and benefits of retirement accumulation options has grown in recent years, persons still need to be concerned with both pre and post-retirement health care due to the potentially devastating financial impact of uncertain health issues. The rising cost of health care works against the ability of the person in attempting to secure their financial future. One means of offsetting both the cost of health care and the related economic risks is to increase the number of persons covered by health insurance. This solution continues to be illusive to government policy makers since 43.4 million Americans representing 16.1 percent of the population of the United States remained uninsured as of 1997 (Kuttner, 1999). Approximately half of the uninsured population is considered low-income, with annual earnings of less than 200 percent of the federal poverty level. These individuals lacking access to preventive and primary care services generally rely on episodic medical treatment that is supported through a number of governmental programs and cross-subsidies from those currently insured (Felland and Lesser, 2000).

Tax Based Approaches To Decreasing Uninsured Rates

The federal government has been providing an estimated $100 billion in tax-based subsidies to encourage increased participation through employer-sponsored health insurance (Gruber and Levitt 2). While the federal government has moved toward increasing the participation of self-employed in the tax subsidized structure, others who are not covered by employer-sponsored plans have been left with minimal tax-subsidized options (Gruber and Levitt 2). Participation in an employer-sponsored insurance program has not come without a negative for the employee. Employers sponsoring the health insurance coverage select the insurance company and the types and amounts of coverage available, many times leaving the employee with little or no choice involving their health care options (Butler and Kendall 2).

While new nationwide survey data from the Center for Studying Health System Change suggest that more consumers have a choice of plans than generally believed, there are variations in plan offerings to families and employees, depending on where the family lives and whether an employee works for a small or large firm. Specifically, the survey findings indicate that only about 55 percent of families living in non-metropolitan and small metropolitan areas who are offered employer-based health coverage have a choice of two or more health plans, compared with 70 percent in large metropolitan areas. Employees in firms of 50 or more workers were also about twice as likely to have a choice of health plan as those in firms of fewer than 50 workers (Trude 3).

Employees participating in an employer-sponsored health insurance program benefit from the ability to exclude the benefit from their taxable income. Amounts received in the form of reimbursements for medical care and payments for the permanent loss of a bodily function are both excludible from gross income (Internal Revenue Code §105). The contributions to the employer sponsored plan by the employer are likewise excluded from the gross income of the employee (Internal Revenue Code §106). When an employee is required to make a contribution to their health insurance cost, the contribution can be made with pre-tax money provided the employer has met the qualifications to do so under the Internal Revenue Code (Internal Revenue Code §125). The result of these benefits is to reduce the cost of the coverage to the employee since none pays tax on the money used to fund the insurance. With the income tax rate on individuals as high as 39.6 percent (Internal Revenue Code §3) and the social security tax rate for the employee and employer at 6.2 percent for each, the savings from these provisions can be considerable. For an employee in the highest tax bracket paying $5,000 for health insurance coverage, a federal government tax subsidy of $2,600 would be received through the exclusion of the health insurance benefit from the income of the employee and the exclusion of the premium from the social security tax paid by the employer and employee.

Congress has addressed the issue of the self-employed by permitting an increasing percentage of the health insurance premium to be deducted from the employees gross income which will provide the insured with a tax-based insurance subsidy (Internal Revenue Code §162(l) as amended by P. L. 105-277). The percentage deductible from the self-employed individual's gross income is based upon the following phase-in percentages:

2000 – 2001:	60%
2002:	70%
2003 and afterwards:	100%

The restrictions placed upon the self-employed are meant to avoid any duplication in tax subsidy. Furthermore, the ability to shop the tax subsidies allows the taxpayer to avail him of herself of that which is most advantageous to his or her individual position. Foremost in the restrictions is the limitation that a self-employed person who is eligible to participate in any other subsidized health insurance plan is not eligible for the deduction in any month in which the eligibility exists. It is also not permitted to take the deduction as both a deduction from the self-employed persons gross income and as an itemized deduction (Internal Revenue Code §213). The deduction is also not permitted to exceed the amount of the individual's net earning from self-employment and, unlike the employee, no reduction in the self-employment income in calculating the self-employment tax liability (Internal Revenue Code §162(l)).

For the Americans who do not receive a tax-subsidized health insurance program though their employers or by virtue of being self-employed, little or no help is available to meet the cost of the health insurance (Butler and Kendall 2). The only tax subsidy available to the individual can be found in the deduction of health insurance premiums as itemized deductions (Internal Revenue Code §213). In order to receive a tax subsidy, the individual must overcome two limitations placed upon the benefit. The amount of the health insurance cost plus all other eligible medical expenses are reduced by 7.5 percent of the individual's adjusted gross income (Internal Revenue Code §213 (a)). Once the allowable medical expenses are calculated, the total itemized deductions must be greater than the allowable standard deduction amount based upon the taxpayer's filing status. For 2000, the basic standard deduction amounts for individuals (adjusted for inflation) are as follows (Internal Revenue Code §63(c)):

Filing Status	Amount
Unmarried Individuals	$4,400
Head of Households	$6,450
Married Individuals Filing Joint Tax Returns	$7,350
Surviving Spouses	$7,350
Married Individuals Filing Separate Tax Returns	$3,675

For a taxpayer with an adjusted gross income of $50,000 and a health insurance premium of $5,000, the 7.5 percent reduction would be $3,750 reducing the allowable medical deduction to $1,250. Without other medical deductions or other itemized deductions the remaining allowable amount would not exceed any of the standard deduction amounts and no tax subsidy to the individual health insurance purchaser.

Employer-Based Coverage Results

While tax subsidies to employers assist with the affordability of coverage, this subsidy has not eliminated the problem of the uninsured worker. The coverage rate of workers -- the percentage of workers insured in firms that offer health benefits -- has actually decreased from 73 percent in 1988 to 67 percent in 1996 with the coverage rate for 1998, 1999 and 2000 averaging 65 percent (Kaiser 43). The coverage rate has also been negatively impacted by the take-up rate, the percentage of eligible workers who choose to participate in health benefits offered by their employer, where the average rate for 2000 was 81 percent (Kaiser 44). The principle reasons cited for not participating included: (1) Having coverage elsewhere, 72 percent; (2) Cannot afford employee share of the premium, 11 percent; (3) Don't want or need coverage, 3 percent; and (4) Don't know or other reasons, 14 percent (Kaiser 51).

The economics of premium sharing with the employee compounds the uninsured rate for the low-income wage earner. The General Accounting Office reports that escalating cost shifting resulted in many lower-income and part-time employees' deciding not to take the health coverage, either for themselves or for their families, because of the cost of insurance coverage (General Accounting Office, 1997). Employers with more than 35 percent of their workers earning less than $20,000 per year pay a lower percentage of the insurance premium than do the employers with high wage levels (Kaiser 73). This differential in benefits is compounded by a shift in co-payments among HMO participants. While for 2000 the majority of workers were paying a $10 co-payment, the percentage declined to 55 percent. This decline was mirrored in the $5 co-payment where the percentage declined to 13 percent. The declines were transferred into an increase in the $15 co-payment to 19 percent, an increase of 9 percent in one year. These factors have a direct impact upon medical services the employee takes advantage of by leading to less utilization of needed services (Kaiser 7)

Health Insurance Portability And Accountability Act Of 1996

The Health Insurance Portability and Accountability Act of 1996, PL 104-191, 8/21/96 was passed by Congress in an effort to make available a more affordable health insurance program which had a long-term benefit of providing an additional retirement savings incentives for those who utilized services prudently. The Act provides for a combination of a high deductible catastrophic insurance plan and savings program through a medical savings account. This new plan would provide individuals the opportunity to accumulate funds tax free to pay for health care costs or, if unused, supplement retirement income (Internal Revenue Code §220).

The medical spending account provides the opportunity for persons to insure against catastrophic health events while functioning in a manner similar to the retirement savings provisions of the Internal Revenue Code. The retirement benefit component of the medial savings account provides the opportunity to assist in creating financial security since funds not spent on health care could be withdrawn penalty-free at retirement (Internal Revenue Code §220(f)(4)(C)). Whether these benefits would reduce the uninsured rate is subject to debate among commentators. The savings feature benefits high-income taxpayers disproportionately while the low-income taxpayer would receive little or no benefit from the provision (Jefferson 704).

Arguments have been advanced that medical savings account eligibility would make it a favored form of insurance for small businesses which currently cover their workers with HMOs (Goldman 71). The basis for claiming a preference is based in the concept of the HMO that prepays a substantial portion of health care costs through the premium. This prepayment provides a substantial tax break to the employee since the premium contributions are tax-exempt while the payment of medical bills is deductible to a limited extent an itemized deduction (Goldman 64). The medical savings account provide the same benefit as the HMO, the contributions to the account are tax-exempt to the employee, while discouraging alleged wasteful spending on unneeded health care (Goldman 65).

The catastrophic insurance concept coupled with the inability of low wage earners to pay the deductible could lead to unwanted risks for such individuals. While the role of the insured would be to become more proactive in their own health choices, the knowledge factor of the medically uneducated individual could cause needed medical care to go unattended with devastating results (Jefferson 718).

Conclusion

A consensus of the literature and research indicates the primary reason for the lack of health insurance among millions of people is the cost of coverage. Most of the uninsured cannot afford to pay for the cost of health insurance premiums which are expected to increase 10 percent or more in 2001 and 2002 (Center of Studying Health System Change, 2000). While assuring access to health insurance coverage (i.e., potential access) to all citizens regardless of their ability to pay is important, health insurance coverage alone does not guarantee utilization of services (i.e., realized access).

Patient co-pays and deductibles appear to be a major financial barrier indicated by one-fourth of the respondents in this study. This barrier is compounded when employers, in an effort to lessen the health insurance cost to themselves, show a trend to increase deductibles and co-pays on the part of the employee. Perhaps local health plans require relatively high co-payments based on national standards, which imposes a significant barrier because of historically lower wages and salaries in the area in which the study was conducted. The transfer of cost to the employee would favor a decrease in any existing over utilization of medical services, yet at the same time creating a barrier to needed services by a portion of the population.

NOTES:

NOTES:

Chapter 8

Marketing

By Cheryl O'Hara

Introduction

The phrase "marketing of health care" is not the oxymoron may people believe it to be. Instead, it is the direction that health care facilities need to move in order to remain viable.

There is a need to move away from the idea that "marketing" is strictly a technique that large corporations use to sell tangible products to consumers. Visions of Willy Loman in "Death of a Salesman" do little to dispel this idea from people's minds. Instead, expansion upon the idea of a "product" needs to include intangible services, such as the providing of health care.

No one argues against the idea that health care is a commodity needed, at least from time to time, by virtually everyone. Therein lies part of the problem – if health care is needed by people, why must the patient be "marketed to"? Why must they be sold on the idea? The fallacy here is that we aren't attempting to convince people to seek out health care. Rather, we want to convince people to seek out health care at our particular facility.

Three factors quickly come to mind that increase the need for marketing a health care facility. First, increased competition from other providers of similar services in the same geographical area dictates that people have a choice of facilities to use. Second, the pressure to fill beds has been exacerbated by the pressure from insurers to shorten hospital stays. Finally, other health care facilities are drastically increasing their marketing efforts, as exhibited through increased advertising and public relations efforts.

Marketing Defined

Clarification of exactly what is meant by the term "marketing" needs to be made. The classic definition is:

Marketing is the process of planning and executing the conception, pricing, promotion, and distribution of ideas, goods, and services to create exchanges that satisfy individual and organizational objectives.[1]

In order for this exchange to take place, at least two different individuals or groups need to be involved. Each needs to have something to offer which is of potential value to the other. How does this work in the health care field? The exchange being considered here is health care services in exchange for monetary considerations (be it cash, insurance reimbursement, etc.). In order for each party to be willing to take part in this exchange, they need to feel that the exchange is balanced. That is, they must feel that what they are giving up is at least equal to what they are getting in return. This is where a potential problem exists. How can an individual put a price on health care?

To deliver this product which is being exchanged, a marketing strategy, or mix of components, must be defined. This marketing mix is a combination of the product/service, pricing, promotion, and location/distribution strategies. These four strategies are interdependent and must be designed in harmony with each other.

In practice, the definition of marketing is further expanded to include the adoption of the "marketing concept." This "marketing concept" provides a framework for implementing a marketing strategy. It is composed of three aspects – meeting the needs of the consumer, meeting the needs of the organization, and integrating the various operating components into a unified whole. It is only when all three components are met that a successful marketing effort can take place.

Mission Statements

Thinking systematically about setting up a marketing plan requires that the organization have a clear Mission Statement. This mission statement must state the business that they are in. An easy response would be "the delivery of health care." However, this same mission statement would then be interchangeable for any health care provider. Rather, thought must go into determining the specific purpose of the particular organization. This is most easily accomplished by using a market orientation. That is, the mission should define the specific market who's needs the organization will meet. This prevents the mission statement from being static – rather, it allows for adaptation to a changing environment over time. With a market orientation,

---

[1]Marketing Research Essential, Third Edition, by Carl McDaniel, Jr. and Roger Gates

the changing needs of the selected market can be met within the framework of the mission statement.

As guidelines, mission statements should be specific, adapted to the surrounding external environment, build upon the organization's unique strengths, and be realistic. Caution should be used in determining the level of specificity. A mission statement that is too broad only speaks in vague, generalized terms about the function of the organization, whereas too narrow a mission statement doesn't allow for changes as the environment surrounding the organization changes. Likewise, the mission statement needs to be contextually placed in the actual environment in which the organization operates. This entails consideration of the needs of the market as well as the strengths and weaknesses of other health care providers in the geographical area. Building upon the organization's strengths means considering what the organization is "good at" – what it does better than any of the competitors. Promoting and building upon this uniqueness will be the focus of the entire marketing plan. Therefore, the mission statement must be carefully crafted to determine future direction. Realism also comes into play. The mission statement needs to motivate those people involved in the organization, which only happens if they feel that the mission statement is workable and attainable.

As an example, the Nashville Metropolitan Bordeaux Hospital states their mission[2] as:

> In accordance with the Charter of Metropolitan Government, and the Metropolitan Hospital Authority Act, the Board of Trustees, the medical staff, and employees are committed to provide quality healthcare services to acutely ill patients of the community in a cost-effective and respectful manner.
>
> Nashville Bordeaux Hospital and Nursing Facility, as the publicly –owned chronic healthcare delivery system, provides long-term care to our patients and the populations served of Nashville Davidson County.
>
> With a commitment to the continuous improvement of quality of all that we do, the staff of the healthcare system shall strive to provide quality, compassionate care and preserve the dignity and quality of life of all patients.

---

[2] http://www.nashville.org/bordeaux/misson.htm

Market Analysis

Prior to considering the specific actions the organization should take to fulfill its mission, information needs to be gathered about the external environment within which the organization exists. Three specific areas should be considered – the target consumers (or clients or patients) to be served, the external environment in which the organization exists, and the nature of existing competition.

For target consumers, the starting point is to identify, in as much detail as possible, who the organization's consumers are. Facts such as their location, age, sex, lifestyle, and income level will all help to clarify exactly who they are. The more that is understood about the specific target market, the better the ability to design and market specific services to them.

Next, information needs to be gathered about any environmental factors that are likely to impact the organization. These are factors that will affect the organization and consumers, but over which the organization has no direct control. Some examples include changes in health care legislation, changes in the health insurance industry, and new directions for patient treatments.

When considering the competition, thought must be given not only to direct competition but also to indirect competition. Indirect competition would include providers of similar services in a different setting. For example, for some services, hospitals compete not only with other hospitals, but also with ambulatory care facilities, same-day surgery centers, and physician's offices. All of these must be analyzed as to their level of competition, considering the uniqueness of how they offer services, their relative pricing (both actual and as perceived by consumers), their location, and their reputation or image in the community.

At this time in the marketing planning process, consideration should be given to how the organization's services compare with those of the competition.

Company Analysis

As part of the analysis process, and before specific goals and objectives can be set, a thorough analysis of the organization must be completed. Some considerations are: physical layout and facilities, finances, asset utilization, image, existing good will, personnel strengths (such as specific skills, innovativeness, and creativity), and the strengths and weaknesses of existing marketing efforts.

144

Upon comparison of the market analysis and the company analysis, it should become clear where the organization has strengths and uniquenesses that can set it apart from the competition. This differential advantage will become the centerpiece of the marketing plan about to be developed. Without a differential advantage, there is no feature that can be used to set the organization apart from the competition in the eye of the consumer.

Marketing Goals and Objectives

Following closely with the mission statement, specific goals and objectives must be set. Whereas the mission statement sets the overall direction for the organization, the goals and objectives set the immediate, short-term direction. These goals and objectives determine the day-to-day operation of the organization, and are used to set specific marketing strategies.

While writing goals and objectives, care must be taken to ensure that they are meaningful, concise, obtainable, and measurable. If the goals and objectives are set at too high a level, thus perceived by those accountable for them as being unobtainable, workers will be demoralized rather than motivated. Stating the goals in measurable terms also helps to motivate people. People will work harder toward meeting goals if they know whether or not they will be able to determine if they have obtained the expected level of achievement.

Marketing Strategy

At this time in the process, the task is to design a comprehensive and coordinated strategy that will achieve the goals and objectives set forth by the organization. Four separate, but synchronized areas must be delineated: product, price, promotion, and location/distribution. Together, these comprise the organization's marketing mix. As opposed to the market analysis, the marketing mix is an area that we can directly control. The organization combines these four marketing tools to produce the desired response from the target market. That is, the marketing mix consists of everything the organization can do to influence the target market to increase their demand for their services.

Product consists of the unique combination of services that the organization is offering to its consumers. The effort here should be to offer services that, as closely as possible, meet the needs of the target consumers. The objective is to offer services that meet their needs more closely than the services offered by the competition.

In today's health care environment, price is an important, but elusive topic. In part, at least, many consumers with adequate health insurance coverage don't feel the need to consider price as an element in their decision as to where to seek health care services. However, as these consumers start to feel the pinch of increased costs for health care coverage, they too will start to consider the price placed on health care services, if only as a means to reducing their premiums.

Promotion encompasses all activities that communicate about the services to the target market. This includes actual advertisements as well as all public relations efforts. Care must be taken as to the message that is being communicated in the promotional efforts.

Whereas it is unrealistic in most situations to think about a total change in location of a hospital, location still plays an important role in the marketing mix. First, location comes under consideration when determining how your expected or desired consumers get to the location. In this respect, consideration needs to be given to topics such as public transportation or safe parking. Whereas safe parking seems far removed in thought from the unique services the facility might offer, consumers concern for safety realistically might cause them to seek care at a different (albeit inferior) facility. Also, location comes under consideration when thinking about satellite or off-site locations for some services. Going to the consumer, instead of the consumer coming to you, is an alternative that should be considered.

Evaluation

Although different organizations use different models to monitor the progress of the business, the important factor is that some mechanism be in place. Quantitative approaches rather than qualitative approaches are considered to be better means of evaluation of the marketing plan. With the use of goals and objectives that have been stated in measurable terms, the evaluation of success has a benchmark system in place. This also helps to motivate the workforce, since results can easily be seen.

Summary

Health care organizations need to continue to push forward with the implementation of marketing strategies. This entails creating a well-planned and integrated marketing plan.

Starting with an evaluation of an existing mission statement, or the creation of a new one, the organization committed to success must consider their differential advantage – how they can serve a particular market of consumers better than the competition. Once they have come to terms with this differential advantage, the organization can then determine how best to market this service to the consumers in an integrated combination of product, price, promotion and location.

NOTES:

148

Chapter 9

Finance and Accounting Issues in Health Care

Dr. David Martin

Review of Financial Statements

Financial Statements are the reports for a business that document its financial health. In a sense, they are analogous to the physical exams one would get from a doctor. There are generally three major accounting statements generated for an organization: The Balance Sheet, Income Statement, and, Statement of Cash Flows. These statements seem different. However, as we shall show, they are interrelated and in total will provide a good picture of the health of the patient, the organization. Let us look at each in turn.

The Balance Sheet

An organization's balance sheet is sometimes referred to as a Statement of Financial Position. It reports accounts balances as of a certain date and, as such, can be thought of as a snapshot of the firm's financial position. The position that is being explored is related to what the organization owns and what it owes, and the difference between the two. The things owned by organizations are called assets. Assets can be tangible or intangible. They can be utilized in a short period of time (current assets), or, over a longer period of time (fixed assets). This distinction between current and fixed assets has important consequences for the Income Statement as we shall see. These items are generally recorded at historical (acquisition) costs, rather than at current market costs. To illustrate this point, imagine you bought your home for $100,000 five years ago. Today, after a market appraisal, the home is thought to be worth $120,000. Accounting rules generally dictate[3] that the Balance Sheet would state the value of the house at its purchased price of $100,000 rather than its present market value of $120,000. A fuller discussion of the implications of this general rule will be had later.

Current Assets

Assets that the organization would consume within a year or so are called current assets. Examples of current assets are:

Cash: coins, currency and bank balances.

---

[3] As in many other parts of life, there are always exceptions to the rule.

Marketable Securities: securities easily converted to cash and not held
for long-term investing.
Accounts Receivables: money owed to the organization by its customers
Inventory: goods that will be consumed in the ongoing operations of the
organization.
Prepaid Expenses: items such as prepaid insurance policies.

Fixed Assets

Assets whose normal consumption occurs over several years are fixed assets.
The asset value is generally reduced over time through a process called
depreciation. We will discuss depreciation more in the Income Statement
section. Examples of fixed assets are:

Property, Plant and Equipment: tangible (real) assets. Examples would
be land[4], MRI's, CT Scanners,
buildings, lab equipment.
Intellectual Property: non-tangible assets which have value. These
include, patents, copyrights, and proprietary
treatments.

Assets are thing the organization owns for the purpose of generating
revenues. But, just as individuals have to use money to acquire personal
assets, so do organizations. That money is supplied by creditors, or, by the
owners of the organization and those amounts are listed on the other side of
the balance sheet equation as Liabilities and Equity. Liabilities are legal
debts that the corporation incurred. They are classified as either short-term
(current) or long-term.

Current Liabilities

Imagine that you borrow $500.00 from a bank to be repaid in 12 months. On
your personal balance sheet that would be considered a current liability. The
same is true for organizations. Current Liabilities are those the organization
would normally pay within one year. Interest to be paid is not generally
included since it is an expense and not a liability. They include:

Accounts Payable: money we owe vendors who have delivered us
services/products on credit.
Notes Payable: short-term bank loans.

---

[4] Land is generally not depreciated since it is not "consumed".

Accrued Wages: wages that have been recognized but not yet paid in cash. Remember that the balance sheet is a snapshot as of a certain date. Assume that an organization pays all its employees on Fridays for all work through Thursday. The end of the fiscal year end falls on Wednesday, Dec. 31, 200X. Employees would have last been paid on Friday, December 24, 200X for work ending Thursday, December 23, 200X. Accrued wages would reflect all that is owed employees for work done on December 24 25, 26, 27, 28, 29, 30, and 31st, 200X .

Accrued Taxes: Taxes recognized but not yet paid.

Current Portion of Long-term Debt: much long-term debt is paid down over time. That portion of principle that the organization expects to pay in the coming year would be listed.

Long-term Liabilities

Debt whose initial maturity is longer than one-year. This section would include:

Term Loans: loans with maturity of over one year to ten years.

Long-Term Debt (Bonds): The maturity (payoff) value of long-term debt.

Capital Leases: the present value of future payments to be made on a capital asset that is leased.

Net Asset Value

Mathematically, this is calculated as the book value of assets – book value of liabilities. Conceptually, however, this represents the summation of undistributed profits since the formation of the organization. This would represent the equity value for a for-profit firm. The importance of Net Asset Value is that any accounting losses suffered by the firm will be charged against this account. Obviously, the larger the amount of this account, the greater the probability the firm will survive in the long-term.

The Income Statement

The Income Statement is also referred to as the Profit and Loss Statement. In pure terms, it represents all revenues minus all expenses, or:

$$Income = Total\ Revenues - Total\ Expenses$$

The Balance Sheet is a snapshot looking at accounts at a particular point in time. In contrast, the Income Statement is a video (flow statement) that captures information for a period of time (usually by month, quarter, and then, by year).

The Income Statement is generally produced on an accrual basis using the matching principle. This means that the expenses of producing revenues are recognized when the revenue is reported, not when they are paid out on cash basis. This means that the Income Statement is not on a cash basis.

Revenues

It is important to recognize that Revenues and Income are not synonymous terms. Revenue represents sales for the firm. For an automobile manufacturer, revenues would represent the summation of the price paid by dealers for each automobile purchased less discounts or returns. For a not-for-profit firm, revenue would be a combination of earned (sales) and contributed (gifted) income. For a hospital, revenue recognized for providing patient services would be earned, and, revenue gained from donations would be contributed.

Operating Expenses

These expenses are those related to producing goods and services central to the core mission of the institution. For example, the cost of the nursing staff for a hospital would be an operating expense for the hospital because nursing activities are generally related to producing patient revenue. If the same hospital suffers a loss on bonds it had purchased for investment activities, that expense (loss) would be a non-operating expense since investment activities are not core to producing patient services.

The type of expenses stated in this section would be salary, wages, benefits, interest, bad-debt expense (unpaid patient accounts) and depreciation and amortization. Depreciation is a non-cash expense that represents the expense of acquiring fixed assets. In other words, the cost of a fixed asset is recognized over time rather than at the point of acquisition. Why? Because the fixed asset will produce revenues over time and we want to match the expense over the time we expect to generate revenues. The presence of depreciation and amortization (which is depreciation for intangible assets) means that Net Income is stated in non-cash terms.

Income From Operations

Income from operations is simply the difference between revenues and operating expenses. An operating profit will be made if the difference is positive, and an operating loss will be made if the difference is negative. The presence of a loss may not be all bad if the loss is less than the non-cash expenses incurred.

Gain/ Loss from Non Operating Income

If we have unusual revenue or expenses (investment income or losses, unusual gifts, gains/losses on the sale of properties) they would be recorded next.

Net Income

Simply the summation/difference between the Income from Operations and Gains/Losses from Non Operating Income. This is the "bottom line" that is so often referred to in the popular press. Simply put, Net Income shows how well the firm has handled its expenses relative to the revenues for the specified time period.

Statement of Cash Flows

The next financial statement we look at is the Statement of Cash Flows that represents the change in the cash account on the balance sheet. To understand this statement we must understand that all organizations operate in a similar fashion. They all raise financial capital (liabilities and equity) in order to purchase assets to conduct operations to return money to the claimants to the organization. What the statement of Cash Flows does is tie the balance sheet and income statement together by recognizing that how money flows into, through, and, out of the organization.

To show the flow of money, the Statement is broken into three parts: Operating Cash Flows, Cash Flows from Investing Activities, and, Financing Cash Flows.

Operating Cash Flows

Generally speaking, the accounting profession recommends that reported Operating Cash Flows come from Net Income adjusted for non-cash expenses and to changes in most to of the current accounts from the balance sheet. Therefore, the first adjustment to Net Income is the addition of depreciation/amortization because they are non-cash expenses. Beyond that, we need to make adjustments for changes in some of the current accounts, or net working capital.

Net working Capital

Net working capital is simply the difference between current assets and current liabilities. Current assets are used in operations to generate additional cash flow. Current liabilities are funding sources for current assets. Therefore, most of these accounts impact operating cash flows. Therefore, we should adjust for changes in operating cash flows based upon whether a change in a net working capital account increases or decreases the cash balance. We will exclude the cash account, obviously since this is what we are analyzing, and the notes payable and current portion of long-term debt since those are considered financing accounts and will be considered later.

To see if we add or subtract an account we ask whether an increase in the book value of the account is a source or use of cash. For example, let us assume that the book value of accounts receivables increases from $1,500 to $2,000. This means that we have granted credit of $500 additional dollars that is a **use** of cash. From this we can easily construct a small table that tell us whether to add or subtract a change in a current asset or current liability account:

Account Change	Source/Use of Cash	Add/Subtract to/from Net Income
Increase in a Current Asset	Use of Cash	Subtract
Decrease in Current Asset	Source of Cash	Add
Increase in Current Liability	Source of Cash	Add
Decrease in Current Liability	Use of Cash	Subtract

When totaled, then, we have total cash flow from operations. Generally, this number should be positive. If it is not, it signals that the organization is unable to finance itself from its continuing operations and is a clear warning that the firm may be heading for financial distress.

Cash Flow from Investing Activities

All organizations buy and sell real assets. This part of the Statement of Cash Flows attempts to adjust the cash balance on the balance sheet for these activities. Further adjustments are made for depreciation so that, again, the total is adjusted to a cash basis.

154

Cash Flow from Financing Activities

In this section, all repayments of debt principle (not interest payments though because they will be counted in Net Income that is part of Operating Cash Flows) for either short-term or long-term will be subjected. Any new borrowings will be added. For-profit firms will deduct any dividends paid, and add any common stock issued.

When these three sections are added we will get the change in the cash account on the balance sheet for the period being reported.

The financial statements give us a picture of where we have been. How we can transform the future is what we will discuss next.

Capital Budgeting

Capital Budgeting is simply the process of determining in which new fixed assets to invest. We are all familiar with buying a car or a new home. The steps we take in deciding to buy a car, or not, is the same as a hospital whether to buy a new magnetic resonance imager. The point to keep in mind is that we use this process to allow us to make decisions today about the way we want to be in the *future*. So, capital budgeting is a major component in the planning managers do to control the future operations of the firm.

Capital Budgeting Process

The process of effective capital budgeting has the following steps:

Searching the Environment

Managers are very good at knowing the internal environment in which they operate. They know what assets are wearing out or need to be more productive. This is a significant part of the capital budgeting process. However, managers must also be very aware of the external environment that will certainly affect future firm performance. For example, what new equipment has been developed that might allow for better patient care? What are competing health organizations doing in building new facilities? What new and interesting equipment is out to better attract the new physicians that they want to better do their job? What new regulations will, or have been, promulgated that will require new disposal methods of medical waste?

155

To search the environment means that managers have to be fully aware of their organization and its fixed assets. They must know what needs to be replaced, and when they will need to be replaced, but they must also recognize the new assets that will be required to remain competitive, meet new laws, and help to attract and retain qualified professional staff.

Creating Options

Once we have decided we might need a new car, we have to understand what our options are. Using the car analogy, potential buyers will ask do we need a vehicle to carry many passengers, or one that gets many miles per gallon? What can we afford and how long will it take to get? What color do we prefer? Two-door, four-door? The process of creating options allows managers to bring as focus to the capital budgeting process. It, if done correctly, also allows managers to better understand the organization in which they work.

Producing Cash Flow Projections

The first principle of producing cash flows is the recognition that we consider only marginal cash flows – cash flows that change because we accept the project. For example, if we purchase a new MRI scanner than the only revenue and expense cash flows for the MRI scanner are considered (with two exceptions). We would not generally consider the cash flows of the radiology department. The first exception deals with the concept of a sunk cost. Suppose we spent $10,000 on a feasibility study for the MRI scanner. We would not consider that $10,000 in the cash flow projection because it will not change if we purchase the MRI or not. In other words, the cost is not a marginal cost.

The other exception is we should recognize any lost of revenue of other revenue producers (cannibalization). If we purchase the MRI scanner, we might find we have less revenue being generated by our CT Scanner. The loss of revenue is a marginal cost and should be factored into our cash flow projections.

Cash flow projections are critical to properly analyze the viability of capital projects. They are calculated simply by producing annual estimates of net income for the project, and only the project, under consideration and then adding back in annual depreciation for the expected life of the project. Once cash flows are established, we can utilize a variety of decision tools in order to determine whether we should proceed with the project, or not.

Utilizing Decision Tools

Given a set of cash flows for the project we are evaluating, we simply need to apply a decision rule to determine the viability of the project. There are three major tools that we can use: The payback period, the internal rate of return, and the net present value.

The payback period is simply the answer to this question: how long does it take the project to recover the investment related to the project? So, if a project requires an investment of $100,000 and we have expected annual cash flows of $50,000 per year for 5 years, the project's payback period will be 2 years ($100,000/$50,000). An acceptable payback period is determined by the firm dependent upon certain factors such as product life cycle, financing cost viability, and the firm's level of risk tolerance.

The net present value is simply the sum of cash flows for the project adjusted for the cost of financing. If the value produced is greater than zero, than the project is acceptable because the value of future cash flows today will be greater than the cost of the investment. If the value is less than zero, the project would not be acceptable because it would not cover the required cost of financing.

The internal rate of return is simply that discount rate that makes the net present value exactly equal to zero. If the calculated rate is less than the hurdle rate for the firm that is the rate of financing) then the project is unacceptable. If the calculated rate is greater than the hurdle rate, the project is acceptable.

If we accept a project, then we should perform one last step: the Audit.

The Audit

After a project's investment has been made and the project revenues are flowing, it is important to audit what has happened. Why? Because successful managers need to know when their decisions have been successful and when they have failed. Both are instructive. The audit should be performed in a way that focuses on whether the process utilized was acceptable, not on the decision-maker's ability to make a correct decision. This is because the decision maker may have made the right decision but an unfortunate result occurred.

If capital budgeting is done correctly, then future income statements and balance sheets will, on average, be positively affected.

Notes:

Chapter 10

Selected Topics
Editorial Addendum

by Dan F. Kopen, M.D.

Having spent the past twenty years as a practitioner in the health care field, and the ten years before that first as a medical student and then as a surgical resident, I have come to recognize a number of issues that will help to determine the future of health care but do not fit comfortably into any chapter in this text. These concepts are drawn from health care economics, third party payer policies, medical education, medical jurisprudence, and the philosophic foundations of medicine. Some of the issues are interrelated while others stand alone as topics for consideration. The subjects are mentioned in an editorial spirit and are not given the more comprehensive scholarly review that authors have given their subject matter in the preceding chapters. The following is an abbreviated summary of several selected issues arranged in an editorial glossary.

Academic Health Centers represent one of the great achievements of 20th century America. A revolution in medical education had begun in the late 1800's and accelerated following the publication of the Flexner Report in 1910. The result was to convert the practice of medicine from a loose business model to a model of professionalism. Based upon three fundamental missions of education, research and patient care, medical schools grew in influence and contribution throughout the 1900's. The reputation of the profession peaked at the time of World War II as a result of the high-profile contributions of the profession, especially medical schools, to the war effort. Cadres of medical faculty were dispatched to provide physician manpower to support Allied troops. The magnitude of the sacrifice was not lost on the public, and medicine was rewarded with increased prestige and support for the profession. Large sums of money were infused into research and huge successes were realized in the development of vaccines, antibiotics, safer surgery (through the development of anesthetics and blood-banking technologies), and public health initiatives. In 1965 a new wave began with the massive infusion of federal dollars in the patient care arena through Medicare. Tremendous technologic advances ensued as entrepreneurs saw opportunities for the application of emerging technologies. Patient care revenue streams came to dominate the revenue sources for the support of medical education. Patient care concerns came to dominate both research and educational objectives of the increasingly bureaucratic medical schools now referred to as academic medical centers. These same revenue streams drove applied science research by private firms and later private-public cooperative arrangements in the health care field. The unintended consequences of unpredicted and uncontrolled growth in Medicare expenditures hit home in the 1980's. Subsequently, the 1990's saw the rapid growth of government encouraged and supported managed care organizations as an attempt to quell the rising tide of expenses. The marked increases in Medicare expenses were in no small part due to the earlier successes in extending the average life span of the population through medical and public health research and federally supported and encouraged increases in the number of allopathic physicians trained on a yearly basis from about 10,800 in 1970 to 17,000 by 1980, where it has remained since that time. By the 1990's the existence of our nation's medical schools had become dependent upon funding sources over which the medical education establishment had little or no control. Prior to the 1990's the medical profession in general, and medical education in particular, had been handsomely rewarded in return for the loss of financial autonomy. There were no losers during the prior decades of abundance as federal and state dollars poured into the health care sector. Now that has changed. Today academic health centers are struggling to keep their missions of education, patient care and research intact and viable. Tuitions at our nation's medical schools have reached such heights that the average indebtedness of graduating medical students exceeds $100,000. Although studies have yet to clearly demonstrate the effects of such a debt burden, there can be little doubt that career choices with respect to specialty and geography as well as discretionary efforts are profoundly impacted. Since 1970 the number of health administrators and managers has grown by a factor of greater than four times the number of physicians at our nation's academic health centers. This is no different that the similar disproportionate growth in bureaucracies in the health care sector outside of medical schools, and the problem needs to be addressed by academic health centers where models of streamlined administrative structures can be developed that may better serve not only their own institutions, but also serve as models for community hospitals and health care systems. Evolving financial tensions are exerting profound effects on medical education. In addition, consumers of health care, both individuals and third party payers, are demanding unrealistic outcomes while forcing medical schools to cope with cost containment strategies that allow neither the time nor the opportunity for students to engage in the lengthy deliberative exchanges that best serve the acquisition of patient care knowledge and skills. As a nation we are allowing one of our proudest achievements of the 20th century to be systematically challenged and harmed. The human capital that is developed through medical education is an asset that offers its greatest returns to society a generation in the future. We can

160

never fully calculate the societal benefits of a healthy academic health center, but we are allowing invaders at the gate to define the financial strategies that will severely impact medical education. Directors at our nation's academic health centers must not succumb to the allures of entrepreneurs and take-over artists who offer the prospect of financial security or support in return for surrender of institutional integrity or control. The academic culture can neither conform to nor satisfactorily mix with the business culture. The mission of an academic center is served through long-range goals and deferred gratification. The academic ethic has been the source of great service to our nation through research, education and patient care and must be preserved through these troubled times in order to remain capable of continuing to serve the future needs of our nation. Ultimately, all health care institutions depend on centers of undergraduate medical education to provide the human capital that makes our community hospitals and other health care systems possible. The boards of community hospitals and other health care systems need to raise their collective voices and demand that the reimbursement strategies that impair the viability of our medical schools be changed to reflect the significant and worthwhile increased costs associated with undergraduate medical education. Over the long term this is in the best interest of all parties in the health care economy, especially our citizens, the ultimate consumers of health care services.

Cherry picking is a well-known phenomenon that many early entrants into managed care availed themselves of in order to gain financial advantage. This consists of selecting a capitated population base on the basis of relative good health. For example, by opening the plan only to defined groups such as actively employed individuals in large clusters an HMO can decrease its aggregate exposure to untoward medical costs. People thus identified have already been selected through work physicals and their ability to continue to work as enjoying better than average health status. By selecting such a capitated audience an HMO provider can offer lower premiums and still increase net revenues. However, this leaves behind for the traditional insurers a less healthy patient base for which they must in turn raise premiums to cover the now higher costs of insuring a less healthy patient population. **Banana scanning** is a related topic whereby an insurer may include in a capitated base persons with certain chronic diseases that can be managed in several ways but will likely require expensive interventions at some point. Implementation of those high-end interventions can often be delayed at the discretion of providers for substantial periods of time. While still unripe, the banana can sit among the capitated base without impacting overall costs. However, as the banana ripens and starts to rot the banana is "encouraged" to change insurance coverage even though the underlying diagnosis remains the same. The new provider, often Medicare or Medicaid,

161

is now saddled with a patient in more urgent need of expensive care. Subsequently, the cost profile of the receiving insurer looks poorer in comparison with the plan that played the game of temporizing on intervention. Medicare has seen many of its HMO plans fail in part as a result of being the insurer of last resort for our nation's elderly and infirm. This effectively precludes wholesale cherry picking or banana scanning. This also renders the traditional insurance products offered by Medicare and Medicaid more reliable and authentic as providers of health care coverage for their defined populations.

Cincinnatus Society is a living example of the "kill the messenger" approach to the uncovering of painful truths. The Physicians' Cincinnatus Society (PCS) was founded in 1986 largely in response to what are felt by many to be unconstitutional burdens of professional liability insurance requirements imposed by Act 111 in Pennsylvania. PCS uncovered evidence in Pennsylvania of a two-tiered system of malpractice insurance premium charges that tilted the playing field heavily against physicians in private practice. Members of this society, standing on principle and acting on behalf of the greater good, have risked and suffered temporary revocation of their licenses to practice as well as having been marginalized by many of the existing powers in the health care field, including the State medical society, in a situation that hints of protective reticence extending beyond individual institutions to include a wide variety of health care and related entities. The very real concerns that have been raised, at a time when the survival of the state's malpractice insurance and catastrophic coverage system is increasingly resting on tenuous grounds, have been largely overlooked and ignored. A system badly in need of overhaul or replacement could benefit greatly by the willingness of all interested parties to take an open and honest look at the findings of this group that has been willing to speak painful truths.

Consumer expectations have assumed greater focus in recent decades. Enormous changes in individual and group expectations occurred during the 20th century. During the first half of the century, both individuals and society viewed health care as a benefit to be purchased at a price that self-reliant individuals and society were willing to pay in the form of out-of-pocket expenditures for individuals and families and philanthropic and governmental subsidies to medical schools and hospitals. Poor medical outcomes were largely attributed to God's will and any benefits derived from health care were for the most part deeply appreciated. By the middle of the century, the expectation of available but unaccountable health care was changing to a belief in a right to health care with a minimal safety net of beneficial outcomes. This belief in a right to health care grew out of a rising expectation that equality of opportunity demanded equal access to at least minimal standards of health services that should not be compromised by financial circumstances. Belief in equal access promoted society's willingness to provide massive infusions of financial resources into medical education and medical care through the "Great Society" initiatives of the Kennedy-Johnson era. Growing expectations soon evolved from the perceived right of equal opportunity of access to the more utopian view of equality of outcome through entitlement. These lofty societal expectations, described by Thomas Sowell as "cosmic justice," have become impossible to achieve under any conceivable allocation of resources in our nation. The accelerating evolution of heightened and impossible expectations is fostered by such diverse interests as our tort system, our civil liberties establishment, our medical advertising industry in service to entrepreneurial initiatives, and our mass media's penchant for reporting attention-grabbing headlines. These have led us to our current predicament of impossible expectations founded on an ethic of instant gratification through entitlements. We cannot satisfactorily address these expectations through central bureaucratic attempts to socially engineer the holy grail of perfect and equal medical outcomes.

Disease management is a concept that has been hailed by some to represent an improvement over the "uncoordinated fracture of care" represented by the typical methods of provision of medical care. This view has arisen from observations of the various levels at which an individual can and often does receive care for a particular diagnosis. These settings include the primary care provider, specialist care providers, outpatient and inpatient diagnostic and treatment venues and non-traditional settings and providers. At first glance it would seem preferable to offer all levels of care for a specific disease at one comprehensive setting. This may prove advantageous for a patient with only one serious illness. However, patients often present with multiple serious diagnoses, and to have each treated through a disease center specific to a particular diagnosis results in what is effectively a "coordinated fracture of care." A patient with multiple serious diagnoses could be caught in the position of having to negotiate between and among various disease centers in search of a balanced approach to general well-being. It is still the case that the vast majority of patients are best served by the care of a knowledgeable, concerned generalist who can, as that patient's advocate, engage appropriate levels of specific expertise in a timely fashion on behalf of his or her patient.

Economies of Scale represent situations in which the average unit cost of production decreases as output increases. This can result from the ability to spread the fixed costs of production across more units as well as the ability to

163

take advantage of reductions in per unit variable costs through bulk purchases and shipping and handling consolidations.

Diseconomies of scale represent situations in which the average cost of production increases as output increases. This can occur when inventories grow beyond efficient carrying capacities, when quality suffers and more defective units are produced, and when the size of bureaucracy stifles innovation and flexibility. There are limits to efficient growth that are particular to each institution, to particular services, and to every catchment area beyond which further growth erodes efficiencies of expansion and economies of scale deteriorate into diseconomies of scale.

Economies of Scope represents situations in which an organization can jointly produce two or more types of goods or services at lower cost than it could separately produce those same goods or services. This makes sense where two types of service draw resources from the same fixed cost pool and can do so efficiently. Economies of scope are not often realized when horizontal integration of services is pursued to acquire control over other providers in the market simply for the sake of expanding a power base.

Diseconomies of scope represent situations in which an organization finds it more costly to jointly produce two or more types of goods or services than it could separately produce those same goods or services. This situation occurs frequently when horizontal mergers and takeovers occur. The failure of leadership to recognize the profound impact of motivational factors on service production often results in both decreased productivity and erosion of the quality of services so acquired. The resultant increases in the unit costs of production and decreased quality under joint production as compared with higher quality under separate process ownership are often unintended consequences of acquisition and consolidation policies in health care.

Health care legislative initiatives represent for the most part well-motivated and honest efforts by interested parties and legislators to improve the health care atmosphere in ultimate service to patients and communities. Groups that represent concentrated interests can and do influence legislation. This has been witnessed in legislative mandates regarding maternity length-of-stays and breast cancer consents to treatment and hospital stays. However, the people trying to pass reasonable health care legislative reforms, and in particular in the field of tort reform, are playing a game in an arena that is only fully understood and most successfully engaged in by lawyers. By far the most successful interest groups have been trial lawyer associations. Not only have lawyers written the rules in jargon that only the legally trained can understand, but they are keenly aware that they hold the trump card.

Lawyers are the almost exclusive possessors of seats on the highest state courts where they wield ultimate authority through judicial discretion to overturn legislative initiatives if they see fit to do so. Depending upon the strength of their belief in judicial activism, justices may be more or less disposed to overrule and/or reinterpret legislative decisions. An overrule by the court occurred in Pennsylvania in 1997. The State Medical Society in 1996 had touted to its membership what appeared to be successful tort reform only to have the legislation gutted by the Pennsylvania State Supreme Court, an action that had been predicted by legal opponents of tort reform even before it had worked its way through the arduous legislative processes. There has been effective usurpation of judicial privilege by the legal profession. Through two centuries of legalism our nation has come to accept the proposition that the only persons qualified to hold offices that decide ultimate secular justice (seats on supreme courts) are members of the bar. Justice and adversarial legalism have become conflated in practice if not in principle. Usurpation of the tort system by trial lawyers has put health care providers and consumers in the unfortunate position of experiencing the tragedy of the commons. The commons of justice need to be recaptured with respect to tort law as it applies to health care. This will then allow full disclosure and search for truth in service to consumers as well as to allow providers of health care to vigorously pursue quality improvement initiatives. It should be noted that in some jurisdictions the most reviled of trial lawyers happen to be honorable practitioners who accept only those cases that clearly meet standards of malpractice and deserve compensation. These few lawyers routinely turn down questionable and nuisance cases. However, the notable successes of these few high-profile malpractice lawyers has created a feeding frenzy among their colleagues that continues to escalate as there is growing recognition that the sources of financial remuneration may soon, and in some cases already have, run dry. In the meantime, human capital in the form of competent and committed physicians is fleeing jurisdictions that allow extreme forms of adversarial legalism to extort large sums of money from honorable and highly qualified providers of health care. Soon, hospitals will be forced to consider the abandonment of their missions as they max out on their catastrophic coverage. Insurers are increasingly reluctant and sometimes refusing to enter markets to provide coverage for those who remain. Studies have shown that professional arbitration boards serve injured consumers in aggregate better than the current tort system. Injured parties fare better with respect to the likelihood of recovery, the timeliness of recovery, and the total dollars actually received by injured parties in aggregate as opposed to the large proportion of judgments that go to pay lawyers' fees, discovery costs, and other friction costs of the tort system. As a board member it is time to get involved in the discussion of tort reform and/or replacement.

Medical necessity is a term used to convey the often misleading assumption that there exists a clear dividing line between health care services that are necessary and those that are not. Furthermore, it conveys an implicit suggestion that such a distinction can be made in real time prior to the full evaluation of the appropriateness of a service and before the provision of that service. In truth, there are at best only varying degrees of likelihood that a service will or will not be medically necessary. In some instances the likelihood may be so high or so low that for practical purposes there appears to be a clear distinction. However, in a large number of instances there is a significant gray zone of uncertainty in which decisions to accept or reject a service should, and by law do, rest with the consumer. The reasons for this large gray zone include the existence of significant variations in disease presentation and severity, variations in susceptibility from person to person, variations in disease definition from culture to culture, and variations within the same person from time to time with respect to any given diagnosis or treatment modality. **Variation**, a biological fact of life driven home to physicians during medical training, is often neither adequately recognized nor appropriately respected by those who would engage in wholesale reengineering of the medical economy and the processes of health care delivery. Some of the most serious misapplications of quality management theories to health care lie in attempts to compel patients and providers to conform to increasingly narrow limits of variation in the provision of services. These progressively more narrowly defined standards of care (e.g. in determinations of length of stay, allowable diagnostic testing, and considerations of therapeutic alternatives, etc.) sometimes disregard the fact that biologic variation cannot be altered by administrative fiat. Attempts to create cookie-cutter approaches to patient management need to be tempered by respect for biology and physiology as well as individual and group preferences among consumers of health care services.

Moral hazard represents the additional amount of health care demanded as a result of the net decrease in out-of-pocket cost of services attributable to insurance coverage of costs for those services. The increased utilization of services under the umbrella of moral hazard is not necessarily inappropriate. For example, this can result in a patient seeking cancer-screening services that lead to detection of a cancer in an early and curable stage. On the other hand it is also be the case that redundant services can be demanded that either add no value to or even harm patient health status.

Immoral hazard is a term I use to denote the reduced amount of health care demanded as a result of the net increase in out-of-pocket cost of services attributable to a decrease or loss of insurance coverage of costs for those services. In today's health care climate this is most keenly experienced by those who have no insurance coverage and who do not qualify for governmental programs of assistance. These individuals are caught in the crossfire between insurers who demand that providers offer deeper discounts, and providers who raise their charges to capture every available dollar in reimbursements. The result is an inflated charge (often double or triple what is accepted as payment from certain insurers) to those who are self-pay patients, effectively driving them away from diagnostic and therapeutic health care services, even at risk to their well being. This is not always inappropriate. For example, this can result in avoidance of adverse side effects of diagnostic and therapeutic interventions that may not have been in the patient's best interests. On the other hand, services that could lead to improved health may be avoided by a patient, ultimately leading to more serious illness.

Nursing shortages are a result of the facts that nurses are overworked, underpaid and not respected.

Optimal demand for health care service is impossible to define. Most commonly this is loosely defined by author/s in a manner to strengthen the apparent statistical power of the conclusions drawn from a study, the conclusions of which are often supported by the definer. Even in the fully capitated environment there will be utilization of services deemed medically unnecessary. Also, in a purely fee-for-service system there will remain among consumers who are fully insured a significant under utilization of medically appropriate and beneficial services.

Patient satisfaction surveys are tools that administrators have learned to manipulate to present only selected information to the board. While useful in concept, a wily administrator can shop for a survey design that will increase the likelihood if not guarantee a favorable report. For example, this can occur when a survey offers five levels of satisfaction to be chosen for a statement wherein three are positive, one is neutral, and only one offers the opportunity to respond negatively. The data collected are often far less important than the wording of the questions asked and the constraints placed on the answers allowed. What really need to be elicited and focused on are responses of dissatisfaction. Unfortunately, the usual practice is to effectively discourage and cover-up negative responses in order to give an inflated representation of patient satisfaction to directors. Whole sections of surveys can be omitted from reports to the board, often hiding vital truths that need attention. Undue emphasis is often placed on insignificant improvement over one reporting period, while rationalizations are offered for substandard or deteriorating performance levels over time. Significant sums of money are spent on these surveys. Too often these surveys are undertaken to comply with regulatory requirements rather than to improve quality. You should insist that these resources be used to the fullest extent possible to discover and speak the truth in ongoing efforts to continuously improve.

Physician-patient relationship is a concept that brings to mind a strong bond of trust and faith in the expertise and advocacy of the physician and the sincerity of the patient in a mutual and total effort to maintain and improve health. Historically this has been protected both by custom and by law from unwarranted intrusions and influences. However, in the increasingly legalistic health care environment there has been significant erosion of this bond. Additionally, through adversarial legalism's ability to dismantle significant portions of individual and public faith in this relationship, as well as the declining respect for patient advocacy inherent in the Hippocratic oath among physicians, this is becoming less a useful model in need of reform and more an anachronism in need of replacement. The heretofore nearly sacrosanct concept of physician-patient confidence may one day be replaced by official and legal acknowledgement of simple contractual arrangements for professional medical services with no guarantees promised. The climate in which medical care is provided has changed dramatically over the past three decades Physicians are often placed in ethical/legal dilemmas that offer no legally correct recourse. As an example, and varying from jurisdiction to jurisdiction, a family physician who provides care for a patient with AIDS can be sued for failure to disclose this diagnosis to the patient's spouse. The same physician who discloses the diagnosis to the patient's spouse, who is also under his care, can be sued by the patient for breach of confidentiality. The frustrations of trying to best serve the health of those entrusting themselves to the physician's care can become overwhelming. Shifting legislative mandates and judicial interpretations do not offer solutions to such ethical/legal dilemmas. The physician's involvement in provision of services and exposure to litigation should be as protected as is the lawyer's in the lawyer-client relationship. This would go a long way towards eliminating the need for tremendous investments of time and energy by health care providers, both physicians and institutions, in protective defensive posturing, thus freeing these resources in service to patients.

Physician over/under supply are terms used to denote either excess of shortage of physician manpower in a defined geographic area during a defined period of time. While the terms sound authoritative in usage, they are seriously flawed when subjected to close scrutiny. Because medical necessity is impossible to define for individuals and populations, the over/under supply of physician providers is also impossible to define.

Furthermore, physician capacity is dependent upon many factors including specialty/generalist mix, utilization of physician extenders and/or replacements, overlap of service areas and physician practice patterns. What has been experienced on a national level has been the wholesale effort to almost double physician supply starting in the mid 1960's by offering financial incentives to medical schools that could not effectively be refused. The result was to nearly double the number of seats available in medical schools. The thought was that by increasing the numbers of physicians health care costs would, through competition, decline. The engineers of that effort must not have had access to the literature regarding supplier-induced demand or any understanding of the tremendous unmet needs of consumers of health care at the time. On a local level, physician supply figures are sometimes bantered about to close medical staffs in order to protect the practices of favorite sons; or, alternatively, to gain support for decisions to hire additional medical staff in selected areas, usually at the behest of favorite sons. In any case, there is little evidence to support the relationship between population health and physician supply. Some of the most under served areas in our nation enjoy relatively good health status while some areas of oversupply are marked by poor health status among the population. What matters most in the poorly understood calculus of physician supply is not the counts of physicians but rather the character of the physicians. A large town containing a few dishonorable physicians is oversupplied while a smaller town having several physicians, each of high ethical standards, is well served. Directors need to be wary of physician supply statistics that are brought before the board in order to influence deliberations. These may simply be ploys to gain unwitting acceptance of hidden agendas.

Statistics are a means of communication that appear to be devoid of emotional overlay and are therefore more likely to be accepted by the unassuming at face value. However, as Mark Twain reminded us in his attribution to Disraeli: "There are three kinds of lies: lies, damn lies, and statistics." Statistics is the language of quality improvement. As with any language, it can be used to manipulate meanings. The often-repeated saying "statistics don't lie, men do," does not paint a realistic picture of the harm that attends the misuse of statistics. Samuel Clemens sounded a warning that has largely been forgotten as we have come to place almost blind faith in statistical presentations without seriously evaluating the methodologies and integrity of data collection and presentation. It is unwise to bestow blind faith in numerical presentations. Numbers alone guarantee neither truth nor objectivity. Furthermore, data can tell half-truths just as words can. Often the half-truth revealed is less important than the half-truth concealed. There are two rules of statistical analysis that come from Walter Shewhart: 1) Data should be presented in such a way that preserves the evidence in the data for all the predictions that might be made from these data (the context should be completely and fully described, a graph should accompany any table, and visa versa). 2) Whenever an average, range or histogram is used to summarize data, the summary should not mislead the user into taking any action that the user would not take if the data were presented in a time series. The time order must be preserved. No data have truthful meaning apart from the context in which the data were collected and transformed. When used ethically and appropriately, statistics offers a powerful tool for the dispassionate analysis of process performance and the search for truth. Directors would be wise to insist that their organizations have an office of statistical analysis that is independent of the administration and reports directly to the board.

Supplier induced demand (SID) is a term used to denote the increase over "optimal" levels in consumer utilization of medical services usually associated with the discretionary influence of providers of health care. Most commonly this is a result of attempts of health care providers to increase profits in fee-for-service plans by increasing utilization of services. The increased service utilization may or may not benefit the patient.

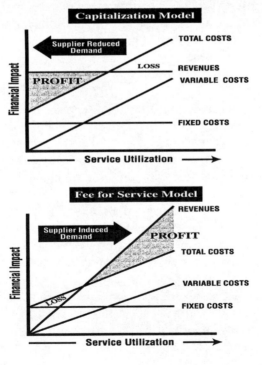

Profit Strategies In Capitated vs. Fee for Service Models

170

Supplier reduced demand (SRD) is a term I use to denote the decrease from "optimal" levels in consumer utilization of medical services resulting from the failure to inform or the discouragement of use of services by the health care provider. Most commonly this is the result of attempts of health care provider to access financial incentives offered by capitated plans in return for reducing the level of use of services among subscribers to the capitated health plan.

Technological imperatives are perceptions among both providers and consumers of health care. The need to "keep up with the Joneses" is such an established part of the health care economy that rational deliberation regarding the acquisition and use of new technologies is nearly impossible. This is manifested not only in the perceived need of providers to offer every new device or procedure, but also in the demands of patients that the latest in technology be applied to them regardless of the appropriateness of the diagnostic or therapeutic modality. What renders the situation difficult to remedy is the fact that sometimes the most unlikely intervention will benefit a patient, and such anecdotal incidents play heavily in building demand for new technologies. With the ranks of suppliers swelling, there is a strong financial incentive to offer new versions of old procedures in an effort to capture market share. On the high end, this is encouraged by manufacturers and providers of health care products through their offerings of expense-paid trips to resorts where "consultative" fees are paid to physician participants for their attendance. Less expensive but more persistent strategies are also employed to gain provider acceptance and increased utilization of new products. Couple this supplier inducement with consumer demand and there is almost no way to prevent inadequately tested technologies from increasing deployment by providers with at best marginal training. The so-called "learning curve" of skill acquisition is a well-described phenomenon that should take place in a lab or under strict supervision, not in clinical practice. At the institutional level, the technological imperative results in the duplication of high-end services that offer attractive reimbursements with concurrent avoidance of services that are poorly reimbursed or must be undertaken at a loss. Witness one small city of approximately 35,000 population with three hospitals, all of which offer cardiac surgical programs, while that same city has no trauma unit. The adversarial cultural bias has so infested our health care institutions that what is good for the community is lost from working memory in the minds of directors and administrators. All this is not meant to imply that technologic advances should be avoided or discouraged. It is not advancing technology that is the problem. Rather, the unrestrained premature use in the clinical setting and the institutional embrace of high end duplicative services are the problems. Financial exigencies almost always trump considerations of what is good for the commons. Insurers and governments, through their policies, seem unable or unwilling to promote the general welfare, probably because the same underlying adversarial culture restricts their abilities to plan or act in a cooperative manner. As a director you should look outside the box of your own institution from time to time to identify community needs and attempt to balance resource allocation to serve the greater good.

Too big to fail is a perverse attitude that has insinuated itself among persons in positions of leadership in the health care economy. This dangerous delusion can occur across the spectrum from small community hospitals (the big boy on the block) to the nation's largest health care conglomerates. This represents an adversarial arrogance that has no place in today's competitive health care marketplace. It serves neither the institution's nor the public's best interests and stands in the way of legitimate attempts to enhance the quality of service to patients. The facts are that at all levels the big boy can and has fallen.

Tort reform is a term used to suggest that the current climate of adversarial legalism peculiar to American jurisprudence has had significant negative unintended consequences on our health care system and that there must be a willingness and ability to change this tort system if health care is to serve our nation's health needs optimally. What is more likely to be effective in the long term is not reform but rather replacement with a different system to compensate those who have had adverse consequences of medical intervention or non-intervention. Serious consideration of no-fault processes of compensation funded through user fees (similar to co-pays and surcharges) arbitrated by combined case-specific expert medical and professional lay panels with administrative judges would go a long way towards providing more just resolutions of adverse outcomes across the population. More frequent, fairer, and fuller compensation to those who have had adverse outcomes have been documented in other nations where less adversarial means of conflict resolution are in practice.

These two-dozen concepts, presented in an editorial spirit, deserve the attention of health care directors. Some of these issues will require broad-based societal initiatives to bring about the changes necessary to improve health care delivery. Others may be addressed effectively within single institutions. Collectively, directors of health care facilities are uniquely positioned to command the attention of policy makers and thereby promote reform and replacement of structures that are encumbering the cooperative pursuit of better health outcomes across our nation.

NOTES:

NOTES:

Conclusion

Health care in the early 21st century will continue to be a field marked by accelerating change. This will present both increasing obstacles to survival and expanding opportunities for growth. Leadership and leadership's understanding of the dynamics of the health care will be critical to the survival of health care organizations. Formally useful assumptions of marketplace stability and safety will no longer pertain as the health care landscape struggles through this period of uncertain transition. Even organizations that have managed to stockpile huge reserves will not remain unthreatened by the forces of transformation.

Service as a director of a health care facility can no longer be viewed as a position of prestige or honor to be passively accepted. We are in the second decade of a torrent of challenges to these institutions of public trust. Chaos and anxiety have replaced stability and safety as descriptors of the health care landscape. Health care directorship entails huge responsibilities to be fully informed and actively involved in the principled and appropriate allocation of scarce resources. Your willingness to forcefully and rationally inquire and to make decisions in an ethical manner will affect the survival of your organization and the well being of the broader community. You must understand that there are both economies and diseconomies of scale. Similarly, you need to have knowledge of both economies and diseconomies of scope.

Changes in the health care economy, the law, technologies, the definition of quality, and consumer expectations have reshaped the health care landscape. Only fully informed and principled leadership will be able to pilot and protect health care institutions during these turbulent times. Chaotic times bring forth the best and the worst in human behaviors. This will hold not only for those impacting your organization from without, but you will also face serious challenges from within as reserves of good will and public trust become embroiled in the turbulent currents of change. What were formally sacrosanct enclaves of public resources such as institutional endowments and capital assets are increasingly viewed as opportunities for personal gain by people who seize upon opportunities during troubled times. Do not let this happen to your community's accumulated good will and public trust. Both legally and ethically you are obliged to serve as a steward of the public trust.

This book is intended to rouse the consciousness of directors of health care and related institutions. It offers neither pabulum nor panacea. Rather, this serves as a challenge to health care directors to take hard looks at themselves as well as their organizations vis-à-vis the serious challenges impacting health care. With the information provided you should be better able to serve the mission of your organization and the well being of your broader community. With added insight you will bring added value to service on the board of your institution. You will be a more effective director, and your organization will be more likely to survive and prosper in service to the health and well being of your community.

References

American Association of Health Plans. (1997). *National Directory of MCOs and Utilization Organization Review*. Washington, DC.

Anderson, G., & Hussey, P.S. (2001). Comparing Health System Performance in OECD Countries. Health Affairs, 20(3), 219-232.

Applbaum, Arthur Isak. (1999). Ethics for Adversaries. New Jersey: Princeton University Press.

Baker, G.R., Natine, I. and Lear, P. (1994). "Organizational Design in Health Care." In the AUPHA Manual of Health Services Management, edited by R. J. Taylor and S. B. Taylor. Gaithersburg, MD: Aspen Publication, Inc.

Beauchamp, Dan E. and Steinbock, Bonnie. (1999). New Ethics for the Public's Health. New York: Oxford University Press.

Becher, E.C., and Chassin, M.R. (2001). Improving Quality, Minimizing Error, Making It Happen; A Five Point Plan and Why We Need It, Health Affairs. May/June 2001, (Online): 13 pages.

Beebe, John. (1992). Integrity in Depth. New York: Fromm International Publishing Corporation.

Black, Henry Campbell. (1979). Black's Law Dictionary. Fifth Edition, St. Paul, Minnesota: West Publishing Co.

Blanchard, Kenneth and Peale, Norman Vincent. (1988) The Power of Ethical Management. New York: William Morrow and Company, Inc.

Blumenthal, D. (1996). Effects of Market Reforms on Doctors and Their Patients. Health Affairs, 15(2), 170-184.

Bodenheimer, T.S., & Grumbach, K. (1996). Capitation or Decapitation. Keeping Your Head in Changing Times. JAMA, 276(13), 1025-1031.

Britz, Galen C., et.al. (2000). Improving Performance Through Statistical Thinking. Milwaukee, Wisconsin: ASQ Quality Press.

Buchanan, J., Goldman, D. and Keeler, E. (2000). *Simulating the Impact of Medical Savings Accounts on Small Business*. HSR: Health Service Research, 35:1, Part 1 (April): 53-75.

Bulger, Ruth Ellen and Reiser, Stanley Joe. (1990). Integrity in Health Care Institutions. Iowa City: University of Iowa Press.

Burns, L.R., Chilingerian, J.A., & Wholey, D.R. (1994). The Effect of Physician Practice Organization on Efficient Utilization of Hospital Resources. Health Services Research, 29(5), 583-603.

Butler, S. and Kendall, D. (1999). *Tax Credits: Expanding Access and Choice for Health Care Consumers through Tax Reform*. Health Affairs (Online), 11 pages. Available: http://web.nexis.com/universe/document?_ansset=GeHavKO-EZYRMsSEZYRUUBR...(2000, Oct.10).

Campbell, C.R., Schmitz, H., & Waller, L. (1998). Financial Management in a Managed Care Environment. New York: Delmar Publishers.

Carter, Stephen L. (1996). Integrity. New York: Basic Books.

Center for Disease Control and Prevention. (2000). *CDC Fact Book 2000/2001* (Online), 91 pages. Available: http://www.cdc.gov/maso/factbook/main/htm. (2000, Oct 15).

Center for Studying Health System Change. (2000). Wall Street Comes to Washington: Market Watchers Evaluate the Health Care System, Issue Brief, 31(September): 1-4.

Charles, C., Gafni, A., and Whelan, T. (1999). Decision-Making in the Physician-Patient Encounter: Revisiting the Shared Treatment Decision-Making Model. Social Science and Medicine, 49: 651-661.

Coile, R.C. (2000). New Century Healthcare: Strategies for Providers, Purchasers, and Plans. Chicago: Health Administration Press.

Coley, C.M., Li, L., Medsger, A.R., Marrie, T.J., Fine, M.J., Kapoor, W.N., Lave, J.R., Detsky, A.S., Weinstein, M.C., and Singer, D.E. (1996). Preferences for Home vs. Hospital Care Among Low-Risk Patients With Community-Acquired Pneumonia. Archives of Internal Medicine, 156(14): 1565-1571.

Conrad, D., Wickizer, T., Maynard, C., Klastorin, T., Lessler, D., et al. (1996). Managing Care, Incentives, and Iinformation: An Explanatory Look Inside the "Black Box" of Hospital Efficiency. Health Services Research, 31(3), 235-259.

Coombs, J.R. (1999). Tying Up Loose Ends, The Three Faces of Quality, American College of Physician Executives Institute.

Copi, Irving M. (1961). Introduction to Logic. New York: The Macmillan Company.

Covey, Stephen R. (1989). The 7 Habits of Highly Effective People. New York: Simon & Shuster.

Covey, Stephen R. (1991). Principle-Centered Leadership. New York: Simon & Shuster.

Daft, R. (2001). The Leadership Experience. Harcourt College Publishers, Philadelphia.

DeAlessi, L. (1983). Property Rights, Transaction Costs, and X-Efficiency: An Essay in Economic Theory. The American Economic Review, 73(1), 64-81.

Deming, W. Edwards. (1982). Out of the Crisis. United States: Massachusetts Institute of Technology Center for Advanced Engineering Study.

Dennett, Daniel C. (1991). Consciousness Explained. Boston: Little, Brown and Company.

Denton, Elizabeth A. (1990). A Spiritual Audit of Corporate America. San Francisco: Jossey-Bass Publishers.

Eddy, D.M. (1990a). Anatomy of a Decision, JAMA, 263(3): 441-443.

Eddy, D.M. (1990b). Practice Policies - What Are They? JAMA, 263(6): 877-880.

Eddy, D.M. (1990c). Practice Policies: Where Do They Come From? JAMA, 263(9): 1265-1275.

Eddy, D.M. (1990d). Designing a Practice Policy: Standards, Guidelines

179

and Options. JAMA, 263(22): 3077-3084.

Etheredge, L., Jones, S.B., & Lewin, L. (1996). What is Driving Health System Change? Health Affairs, 15(4), 93-104.

Evidence Based Medicine Working Group. (1992). Evidence Based Medicine: A New Approach to Teaching the Practice Of Medicine. JAMA, 268(17): 2420-2425.

Feldstein, P.J. (1985-86). Productivity and Effectiveness: An Economist's Viewpoint. Health Matrix, 3(4), 19-23.

Feldstein, P.J. (1999). Health Policy Issues: An Economic Perspective on Health Reform. Second edition. Chicago: Health Administration Press.

Felland, L.E., and Lesser, C.S. (2000). "Local Innovations Provide Managed Care For The Uninsured." *Center for Studying Health System Change Issue Brief*, 25(January): 1-6.

Fizel, J.L., & Nunnikhoven, T.S. (1992). Technical Efficiency of For-Profit and Non-Profit Nursing Homes. Managerial and Decision Economics, 13, 429-439.

Fizel, J.L., & Nunnikhoven, T.S. (1993). The Efficiency of Nursing Home Chains. Applied Economics, 25, 49-55.

Flexner, Abraham. (1960). The Flexner Report. New York: Sourcebook

Series, (reproduced).

Folland, Goodman Stano. (1997). The Economics of Health and Health Care. New Jersey: Prentice Hall.

Frantz, R. (1985). X-Efficiency Theory and its Critics. Quarterly Review of Economics and Business, 25(4), 38-58.

Frech, H.E., III. (1976). The Property Rights Theory of the Firm: Empirical Results from a Natural Experiment. Journal of Political Economy, 84, 143-152.

Fukuyama, Francis. (1995). Trust. United States: Simon and Schuster.

Gabel, J.R., Levitt, L., Pickreign, J., Whitmore, H., Holve, E. Hawkings, S., & Miller, N. (2000). Job-Based Health Insurance in 2000: Premiums Rose Sharply While Coverage Grows. Health Affairs, 19(5), 144-151.

General Accounting Office. (1997). *Employment-based Health Insurance: Costs Increase and Family Coverage Decreases.* Washington, D.C.: Government Printing Office, 2(February), (GAO/HEHS-97-35).

Ginsburg, P.B. (2001). Analyzing the changing health system: The path taken and the road beyond. Health System Change Annual Report 2000. Washington DC.: Center for Studying Health System Change.

Ginsburg, P.B., & Lesser, C.S. (2001). Understanding Health System Change: Local Markets, National Trends. Chicago: Health Administration Press.

Glandon, G.L., & Morrisey, M.A. (1986). Redefining the Hospital-Physician Relationship Under Prospective Payment. Inquiry, 23, 166-175.

Gold, M., & others. (1995). Arrangements Between Managed Care Plans and Physicians: Results from a 1994 Survey of Managed Care Plans. Washington, D.C.: Mathematical Policy Research.

Goldman, F., & Grossman, M. (1983). The Production and Cost of Ambulatory Medical Care in Community Health Centers. Advances in Health Economics and Health Services Research, 4, 1-56.

Goleman, Daniel. (1985). Vital Lies, Simple Truths. New York: Simon and Schuster.

Grieco, P.J. & Eisenberg, J.M. (1993, October 1). Changing Physician Practices. New England Journal of Medicine, 329(17), 1271-1273.

Grimshaw, J.M. and Russell, I.T. (1993). Effect of Clinical Guidelines on Medical Practice: A Systematic Review of Rigorous Evaluations. Lancet, 342(8883), (Online): 1317-1323.

Gruber, J. and Levitt, L. (2000). *Tax Subsidies for Health Insurance: Costs and Benefits.* Health Affairs (Online), 10 pages. Available: http://web.nexis.com/universe/document?_ansset=GeHavKO-EZYRMsSEZYRUUBR...(2000, Oct.10).

Hammer, M. (1998). Beyond Reengineering. Harper Business.

HCFA web site. (2001). www.hcfa.gov/medicaid/trends00.pdf.

HCFA web site. (2001). www.hcfa.gov/stats/35chartbk.pdf.

HCFA web site. (2001). www.hcfa.gov/stats/nhe-oact/hilites.htm.

Heizer, J., and Render, B. (1996). Production and Operations Management. Prentice Hall, Inc.

Hellinger, F.J. (1996). The Impact of Financial Incentives on Physician Behavior in Managed Care Plans: A Review of the Evidence. Medical Care Research & Review, 53(3), 294-314.

Hillman, A.L. (1991). Managing the Physicians: Rules versus Incentives. Health Affairs, Winter, 138-191.

Hillman, A.L., Pauly, M.V., Kerstein, J.J. (1989). How do Financial Incentives Affect Physicians' Clinical Decisions and the Financial Performance of Health Maintenance Organizations? New England Journal of Medicine, 321, 86-92.

Himmelfarb, Gertrude. (1995) The De-moralization of Society. New York: Alfred A. Knopf.

Hughes, J.M. (1998). The Cost of Poor Quality: An Opportunity of Enormous Proportions. Physician Executive, 24(5), (Online): 46-52.

Institute of Medicine. (2000). To Error is Human: Building a Safer Health System. National Academy Press.

James, B. (1993). Implementing Practice Guidelines through Clinical Quality Improvement. Frontiers of Health Services Management, 10(1): 3-35.

Jefferson, R. (1999). *Medical Savings Accounts: Windfalls for the Healthy, Wealthy and Wise.* Catholic University Law Review, 685.48 (Online), 38 pages. Available: http://web.nexis.com (2000, Oct.21).

Jensen, N. (1999). How Evidence-based Medicine Incorporates Patient Preferences. Wisconsin Medical Journal, March/April: 49-52.

Johnson, Oliver A. (1965). Ethics. New York: Holt, Rinehart, and Winston.

Kagan, Robert A. (2001). Adversarial Legalism. Cambridge, Massachusetts: Harvard University Press.

Kaiser Family Foundation and Health Research and Educational Trust. (2000). *Employer Health Benefits 2000 Annual Survey.*

Karlson, E.W., Daltroy, L.H., Liang, M.H., Easton, H.E., and Katz, J.N. (1997). Gender Differences in Patient Preferences May Underlie Differential Utilization of Elective Surgery. American Journal of Medicine, 102(6): 524-530.

Kleinsorge, I.K., & Karney, D.F. (1992). Management of Nursing Homes Using Data Envelopment Analysis. Socio-Econ. Plan Sci., 26(1), 57-71.

Knight, W. (1998). Managed Care: What it is and How it Works. Maryland: Aspen Publishers, Inc.

Kongstvedt, P.R. (2001). Essentials of Managed Care. Fourth Edition. Maryland: Aspen Publishers, Inc.

Kopen, Pamela A. (1993). Trillium Trail. Padakami Press.

Kotter, J. & Heskett, J. (1992). Corporate Culture and Performance. Free Press.

Kotter, J. (1995). The New Rules. Free Press.

Kravitz, R.L., Callahan, E.J., Paterniti, D., Antonius, D., Dunham, M., and Charles, E. (1996). Prevalence and Sources of Patients' Unmet Expectations. Annals of Internal Medicine, 125(9), (Online): 730-737.

Kuratko, D., and Welsch, H. (2001). Strategic Entrepreneurial Growth. Harcourt, Inc.

Kuttner, R. (1999). "The American Health Care System, Health Insurance Coverage." *The New England Journal of Medicine*, 340(2): 163-168.

Kwon, S. (1996). Structure of Financial Incentive Systems for Providers in Managed Care plans. Medical Care Research and Review, 53(2), 149-161.

Lee, R.H. (2000). Economics for Healthcare Managers. Chicago: Health Administration Press.

Leibenstein, H. (1980). Inflation, Income Distribution and X-Efficiency Theory. London, England: Croom Helm.

Lesser, C.S., & Brewster, L.R. (2001). Chapter 2: Hospital Mergers and Their Impact on Local Communities. In Ginsburg, P.B., & Lesser, C.S. (Eds.). Understanding Health System Change: Local Markets, National Trends. (pp. 19-36). Chicago: Health Administration Press.

Lesser, C.S., & Ginsburg, P.B. (2000). Update on the Nation's Health Care System: 1997-1999. Health Affairs, 19(6), 206-216.

Ludmerer, Kenneth M. (1999). Time To Heal. New York: Oxford University Press.

Lundberg, George D. (2000). Severed Trust. United States: Basic Books.

Lutz, J.A., and Shaman, H.J. (2001). The Impact of Consumerism on Managed Care in Kongstvedt, P.R., eds. Essentials of Managed Health Care: 566-585.
Miller, R.H., & Luft, H.S. (1997). Managed Care: Past Evidence and Potential Trends. Frontiers of Health Services Management, 9(3), 3-37.

Morrison, I. (2000). Health Care in the New Millennium: Vision, Values, and Leadership. Jossey-Bass Publishers, San Francisco.

Nash, D. (1999). Introduction to Clinical Practice Guidelines, The Three Faces of Quality. American College of Physician Executives Institute.

Niskanen, W.A. (1968). Nonmarket Decision Making. The Peculiar Economics of Bureaucracy. American Economic Review, 58, 293-305.

Norretranders, Tor. (1998). The User Illusion. New York: Viking.

Nyberg, David. (1993). The Varnished Truth. Chicago: The University of Chicago Press.

Ogden, D., Carlson, R., & Bernstein, G. (1990). The Effect of Primary Care Incentives. Proc. 1990 Group Health Institute. Washington, DC: Group Health Association of America.

Owen, D.K. (1998). Patient Preferences and the Development of Practice Guidelines. SPINE, 23(9): 073-1079.

Pellegrino, Edmund D. (1979). Humanism and the Physician. Knoxville: The University of Tennessee Press.

Pellegrino, Edmund D. and Thomasma, David C. (1981). A Philosophical Basis of Medical Practice. New York: Oxford University Press.

Phelps, C.E., and Mooney, C. (1992). Correction and Update on "Priority Setting in Medical Technology Assessment". Medical Care, 30: 744-751.

Pindyck, R.S., & Rubinfeld, D.L. (1989). Microeconomics. New York: Macmillan.

Pinker, Steven. (1997). How the Mind Works. New York: W. W. Norton & Company.

Pointer, D.D., Alexander, J.A., & Zuckerman, H.S. (1995). The Governance Challenge: Preserving Community Mission with Integrated Health Systems. Frontiers of Health Services Management, 11(3), 9-10.

Ramachandran, V.S. and Blakeslee, Sandra. (1998). Phantoms in the Brain. New York: William Morrow and Company, Inc.

Reagan, M.D. (1987). Toward Full Disclosure of Referral Restrictions and Financial Incentives by Prepaid Plans. New England Journal of Medicine, 317, 1729-1734.

Reynolds, R.A., Rizzo, J.A., and Gonzalez, M.L., (1987). The Cost of Medical Professional Liability. JAMA, 257(20): 2776-2781.

Rice, T. (1997). Physician Payment Policies: Impacts and Implications. Annual Review of Public Health, 18, 549-65.

Ridley, Matt. (1997). The Origins of Virtue. New York: Penguin Books.

Robbins, Stephen P. (2000). Essentials of Organizational Behavior. New Jersey: Prentice Hall.

Rosko, M.D., Chilingerian, J.A., Zinn, J.S., & Aaronson, W.E. (1995). The Effects of Ownership, Operating Environment, and Strategic Choices on Nursing Home Efficiency. Medical Care, 33(10), 1001-1021.

Schecter, A.D., Goldsmith-Clermont, P.J., McKee, G., Hoffeld, D., Myers, M., Velez, R., Duran, J., Schulman, S.P., Chandra, N.G. (1996). Influence of Gender, Race and Education on Patient Preferences and Receipt of Cardiac Catherizations Among Coronary Care Unit Patients, The American Journal of Cardiology, 78(9): 996-1001.

Schmitt, Frederick F. (1995). Truth, A Primer. Boulder: Westview Press.

Seligman, Adam B. (1997). The Problem of Trust. New Jersey: Princeton University Press.

Senge, Peter M. (1990). The Fifth Discipline. New York: Doubleday Currency.

Shekelle, P.G., Kahan, J.P., et al. (1998). The Reproducibility of a Method to Identify Overuse and Underuse of Medical Procedures. New England Journal of Medicine, 338(26): 1888-1826.

Shelton, Ken (editor). (1998). Integrity at Work. Chicago: Executive Excellence Publishing.

Sherbourne, C.D., Strum, R., and Wells, K.B., (1999). What Outcomes Matter to Patients. Journal of General Internal Medicine, 14: 357-363.

Short, A.C., Mays, G.P., & Lake, T.K. (2001). Provider Network Instability: Implications for Choice, Costs, and Continuity of Care. Issue Brief No. 39, Center for Studying Health System Change. Washington, DC., June.

Siegel, E.R., Cummings, M.M., and Woodsmall, R.M. (1990) Bibliographic-Retrieval Systems in Shortliffe, E.H., and Perrault, L.E., eds. Medical Informatics: Computer Applications in Health Care: 435.

Stearns, S.C., Wolfe, B.L., & Kindig, D.A. (1992). Physician Response to Fee-for-Service and Capitation Payment. Inquiry, 29, 416-425.

Stiggelbout, A.M., and Kiebert, G.M. (1997). A Role for the Sick: Patient Preferences Regarding Information and Participation in Clinical

Decision-making. Canadian Medical Association Journal, 157(4), (Online): 383-389.

Todaro, T. and Schott-Baer, D. (2000). Plan Faster, Healthier Recovery after Orthopedic Surgery. Nursing Communities, 31(1): 24-26.

Trude, S. (2000). "Who Has A Choice Of Health Plans?" *Center for Studying Health System Change Issue Brief*, 27(February): 1-4.

Tuckman, H. P., & Chang, C.F. (1988). Cost Convergence Between For-Profit and Not-for-Profit Nursing Homes: Does Competition Matter? Quarterly Review of Economics and Business, 28, 50-65.

Valiela, Ivan. (2001). Doing Science. New York: Oxford University Press.

Vickery, D.M., and Lynch, W.D. (1997). Patient Expectations and Demand Management, Annals of Internal Medicine, 126(9), (Online): 744.

Wachtel, T.J., & Stein, M.C. (1993). Fee-for-Time System: A Conceptual Framework for an Incentive-Neutral Method of Physician Payment. JAMA, 270(10), 1226-1229.

Walton, Douglas N. (1989). Informal Logic. Cambridge, U.K.: Cambridge University Press.

Weeks, J.C., Cook, E.F., O'Day, S.J., Peterson, L.M., Wenger, N., Reding, D., Harrell, F.E., Kussin, P., Dawson, N.V., Connors, A.F., Lynn, J., and Phillips, R.S. (1998). Relationship Between Cancer Patients' Predictions of Prognosis and Their Treatment Preferences. JAMA, 279(21), (Online): 1709-1714.

Wennberg, J.E., and Gittlesohn, A. (1973). Small Are Variations in Health Care Delivery. Science, 182: 1102-1108.

Wennberg, J.E., and Gittlesohn, A. (1982). Variations in Medical Care Among Small Areas. Scientific American, 246: 120-134.

Wennberg, J.E., Frecman, J.L., Shelton, R.M., and Bubolz, T.A. (1989). Hospital Use and Mortality Among Medicare Beneficiaries in Boston and New Haven. New England Journal of Medicine, 321(17): 1168-1173.

Williams, S.J., & Torrens, P.R. (1999). Introduction to Health Services, (5th Ed.). New York: Delmar Publishers.

Zuckerman, S. (1984). Medical Malpractice: Claims, Legal Costs and the Practice of Defensive Medicine. Health Affairs, 3(3): 128-133.

Glossary

Ad Hominem: An argument or appeal based on attacking the person rather than truth or logical cogency of the person's argument; *abusive* form attacks the character of the man, *circumstantial* form attacks the situation the man occupies, i.e. the relationship between a person's beliefs and his circumstances.

Adjusted Gross Income: An individual taxpayers gross income reduced by certain income tax deductions, such as, contributions to individual retirement accounts, alimony payments, student loan interest deductions, moving expenses, etc. These deductions are not included in a taxpayers itemized deductions which are calculated separately.

Appeal to Authority: (*argumentum ad verecundiam*) An argument based on the feeling of respect for the famous or of an expert outside of that expert's field of expertise rather than on the merits of truth or logical cogency.

Appeal to Force: (*argumentum ad baculum*) An argument based on force or the threat of force to cause acceptance of a conclusion, the "might makes right" approach to gaining acceptance of one's proposals.

Appeal to Pity: (*argumentum ad misericordiam*) An appeal to pity for the sake of getting a conclusion accepted.

Appeal to Populus: (*argumentum ad populum*) An attempt to win assent to a conclusion by rousing the feelings and enthusiasms of the multitude; the bandwagon appeal, i.e. everyone else is doing it, why shouldn't we.

Argument by Accident: The acceptance of a claim on the basis of applying a generalization to a specific case in which the circumstances make the generalization inapplicable; the converse of hasty generalization.

Argument from Adverse Consequences: Using the threat, either explicit or implicit, of unfavorable consequences to deflect consideration away from the truth of a proposal or statement.

Argument from Ignorance: (*argumentum ad ignorantiam*) An attempt to gain acceptance of a claim just because it has not been proven false or, conversely, an attempt to secure rejection of a claim just because it has not been proven true.

Automatism: The deletion of a portion of what is perceived from awareness extending to include the response one makes to that which is selectively intended to.

Balance Sheet: A financial statement that shows the value of assets which must equal the value of liabilities and equity.

Begging the Question: (*petitio principii*) i.e., Assuming as a premise for one's argument the very same conclusion one intends to prove; assuming the answer in the formulation of a proposition; also referred to as the circular argument.

Black and White Fallacy: A fallacy committed when requiring a pair of terms to exhaust a relevant class of objects or states of affairs without residue and when in fact the pair of terms do not exhaust the class. A common example is the statement "If you are not 100% for me then you are against me" or "if you are not 100% against him then you are for me."

Capital Budgeting: A process by which fixed assets are acquired.

Carve Out: Refers to a defined set of health care services (e.g., behavioral health) that are excluded from a basic covered care under a health insurance plan and contracted out to a separate organization or vendor (e.g., a behavioral managed healthcare organization).

Cause and Effect Diagram: Used to produce a comprehensive set of potential causes for an identified performance problem by grouping the potential sources of poor performance into major classifications and then refining these into specific factors.

Complex Question: A fallacy committed when a plurality of questions is undetected and a single answer is demanded which commits the respondent to accepting the premises implied by the hidden questions. The prototypical complex question is "Have you stopped beating your wife?" This is actually three questions: 1) Do you have a wife? 2) If the answer to #1 is affirmative, then are you or have you ever beaten your wife? 3) If the answer to both #1 and #2 are affirmative, then have you stopped beating your wife?

Confusion of Correlation with Causation: The unjustified argument that concludes that one event causes another simply because there is a positive correlation between the two events; the crowing of the rooster does not cause the sun to rise.

Consumerism: The idea that patients should not only receive an explanation of what treatments are contemplated and the possible outcomes but be offered an active role in selecting treatments. Consumerism challenges health care providers to modify health delivery processes to meet the medical and non-medical concerns of patients i.e. convenience, access and cost.

Control Charts: Used to examine the performance of a system, its central tendency and variability, based on upper and lower limits within which performance can fluctuate before investigation and correction is undertaken.

Culture: The pattern of behavior or style that is predominant in the place of work.

Current Assets: Short-tem assets that are easily convertible to cash.

Current Liabilities: Debts that will be payable within a year.

Deferred Tax Liability: Postponement of taxes from one tax year until a later tax year.

Denial: The refusal to accept things as they are; realigning the facts to obscure the actual case.

Employee Development: Any activity that is intended to help prepare the employee for future jobs or future tasks.

Employee Productivity: Refers to any indicator of employee performance, including performance appraisal scores, units produced, number of sales, etc.

Empowerment: The total sharing of power with followers.

Evidence Based Medicine: Stresses the need to base treatment plans on the examination of evidence from clinical research and de-emphasizes the use of intuition, unsystematic clinical experience, and pathophysiologic rationale as sufficient grounds for clinical decision making.

Expatriate: An employee from the country in which the company is headquartered who is reassigned to a job for the company that is located in another country.

Extended Middle: A fallacy committed wherein the objects or states of affairs that are neither black nor white are all considered to be the same; e.g., the 5th and the 95th rated performances are the same as neither was first nor last, i.e., they are both part if the (extended) middle.

False Alternatives: A fallacy committed when only two options are allowed to be considered when in truth other options exist and are relevant for consideration.

False Cause: An attempt to argue on the basis of a causal relationship that is not true; often a mistake of correlation or of timing with causation.

Fixed Assets: Long-term assets that are either depreciated or amortized over time.

Flextime: A system that allows employees the flexibility to vary their starting and ending times for a given workday.

Followership: Consists of dedicated supporters who agree with the leader's vision.

Global Capitation: Represents a single capitation payment made by a health insurance plan to a health care institution that is responsible for the full scope of medical care services (e.g., institutional and professional) to be provided to the covered members of the health plan.

Good Person Fallacy: An argument that if a person does something good, then that person must be a good person; a failure to see the distinction between actions and persons. The Bad person fallacy is committed when arguing that if a person does something bad, then that person must be a bad person.

Gross Income: Total income of a business or individual taxpayer which is subject to taxation.

Half-Truth: An argument that is supported by suppressing evidence and only revealing parts of the whole truth to emerge; a common and virulent form of truth decay that is particularly effective in disarming our neurological lie-detecting abilities and disabling the ability to objectively seek truth.

Hasty Generalization: A fallacy of accepting a generalization on the basis of instances that do not constitute a fair sample; the converse of the fallacy of accident (wherein a general rule is applied to a particular case in which the rule is inapplicable).

Headhunters: Refers to recruiters that target the leaders (heads) of other companies and tries to persuade them to move to other companies.

Horizontal Consolidation: The coordination or consolidation of facilities or services that are at the same stage of the patient care production process to reduce redundancies or duplication of services and also to achieve economies of scale.

Inappropriate Care: Over or under-use of medical services that produces no health benefit for a patient or subjects the patient to unnecessary risks.

Income Statement: A financial statement that expresses the net income of the firm as total revenues minus total expenses.

Internal Revenue Code: Title 26 of the United States Code, the body of laws which codifies all the laws regarding the federal taxation of income, deductions, estates, gifts, etc. Due to extensive changes to the tax law in that year, the common name in Internal Revenue Code of 1986.

Inconsistency: An argument in which the premises are inconsistent (wherein two or more premises cannot be true) and as a result it cannot be a sound argument and no conclusion can be established as true.

Intranet: An electronic internal network accessible to employees that contains information and resources pertinent to the organization.

Irrelevant Conclusion: (*ignoratio elenchi*) A fallacy of ignoring the issue when an argument fails to prove the conclusion it is supposed to prove and instead is directed at proving an irrelevant conclusion.

Isolation: While not repressing an unpleasant event, the feelings it evokes are blanked out of experience; the facts remain with no feelings attached.

Itemized Deductions: Certain personal deductions which are allowed by the Internal Revenue Code as deductions from a taxpayers adjusted gross income. A taxpayer can choose between using a standard deduction amount or itemized deductions. Examples of itemized deductions are state and local income tax, charitable contributions, mortgage interest, certain medical costs and casualty losses.

Job Design: Refers to various methods of changing job requirements, task procedures or the work environment with the intent of improving the employee's job efficiency or effectiveness.

Job Enrichment: A job design technique that attempts to make jobs more rewarding and meaningful through actions such as increase variety or autonomy on the job.

Keogh Plans: Retirement plans available only to self-employed persons which are also referred to as H.R. 10 plans. Contributions to such plans are deductible from gross income of the individual taxpayer in computation of adjusted gross income.

Learning Organization: Individuals are designed for learning. A learning organization encourages learning and increasing adaptability of its employees.

Long-Term Liabilities: Debts whose original maturity are longer than one year.

Marketing Concept: The philosophy that achieving organizational goals depends on determining the needs and wants of target markets and delivering the desired satisfactions better and more efficiently than the competition

Marketing Mix: The combination of product/service, price, location/distribution, and promotion that the organization blends to produce the response it wants from the target market

Marketing Strategy: The logic by which the organization hopes to achieve its marketing objectives

Meaningless Question: The introduction of a question devoid of substance or relevance to the argument in an effort to thwart the process of proposition development.

Medical Decision-Making: The determination of a treatment plan for a patient based on an analysis of treatment options and understanding of the patient's preferences for each option and the outcomes it produces.

Medical Paternalism: The belief that medical decision making should be overwhelmingly the responsibility of physicians due to the nature of medical science and that the physician's information advantage and concern for patient welfare will ensure that optimal treatments are selected.

Naturalistic Fallacy: The mistake of equating what *is* with what *ought* to be; conflating the existence of a procedure with what is morally or ethically the proper procedure.

Net Asset Value: Representation of the equity value of a not-for-profit firm.

Networking Capital: Current assets minus current liabilities.

Non-Sequitur: An inference that does not follow from the premises; the fallacy of drawing a conclusion from premises that do not allow for the conclusion to be drawn.

Observational Selection: The use of ordinary concepts and inferences of observed phenomena places limits to the upper bound of generality that can be attained; mistakenly believing that what has been observed represents either the whole of the range of reality or a true representation of the frequency and severity of occurrence of reality.

Patient Preferences: Attitudes of a patient towards medical treatments and potential outcomes.

Patient Rights: Legally recognized standards that providers must meet to ensure that patients understand and concur with their treatment including the right of informed consent and the right to decline treatment.

Physician/Hospital Organization (PHO): A separate legal entity that represents both a hospital and a physician organization and is empowered to negotiate or contract with health plans on behalf of both the hospital and the physicians.

Plan-Do-Check-Act (PDCA) Cycle: A trial and learning model designed to reduce variation and continuously improve quality involving establishing benchmarks, determining where improvements can be made and implementing changes, evaluating the impact of these changes and implementing further changes based on the knowledge gained through the PDCA process.

Post Hoc Ergo Propter Hoc: A fallacy that concludes that one of two correlated events causes another simply because the one event precedes the other in time; an example of mistaking correlation with causation.

Power: The ability to influence individuals to obtain chosen goals. The base of power can originate from the position and would include: legitimate, reward and coercive elements. Power may also reside within the individual and would include: expertise and charismatic dimensions.

Practice Policies: The delineation of what services should be rendered to a patient. Practice policies range from standards, rigid guides that should be followed in all cases, to options, which simply present alternatives and do not recommend any particular intervention.

Premium Sharing: When an employer requires an employee to pay a portion of the cost of insurance as a condition of the employees participation in the insurance plan.

Projection: This consists first in blocking an unpleasant truth from awareness and then displacing the feelings evoked outward onto someone else.

Quality Management Program: A management system designed to ensure the delivery of optimal care. A quality management program requires the setting of measurable and relevant goals, monitoring performance and feedback to health care providers.

Rationalization: Lies that are so cloaked with reasonableness that we are able to tell them to ourselves as well as to others without flinching; commonplace strategies of convincing excuses and alibis.

Repression: Keeping a thought from awareness; forgetting and then forgetting that one has forgotten.

Reversal: Denial of fact and then transforming the fact into its opposite; sometimes called reaction formation.

Risk Pool: The aggregation of capitation withholds and other incentive or bonus payments that are initially withheld to be redistributed to providers at a later date only if predetermined goals are met.

Roth IRA: Named for its Congressional sponsor, Senator William Roth of Delaware, the IRA permits non-tax deductible contributions, subject to certain limits, and the withdrawal of the contributions and the earnings on such contributions are not subject to federal income taxation if the withdrawal occurs after the taxpayer reaches a prescribed age.

Selective Inattention: The editing from conscious experience those elements that would be painful or unpleasant if noticed; probably the most common psychological defense mechanism.

Six-Sigma: Establishes a goal of 3.4 product failures for every 1,000,000 products produced.

Special Pleading: An argument or presentation that omits what is unfavorable and develops only what is favorable to the case.

Statement of Cash Flows: A financial statement that analyzes the change in the cash account on the balance sheet by analyzing activity in Operating Cash Flows, Investing Cash Flows, and Financing Cash Flows.

Statistical Process Control: The application of statistical techniques to determine when a process is operating up to expectations (in-control) and when adjustments must be made to meet standards (out-of-control).

Stop-Loss Insurance: A form of reinsurance purchased by a health care plan or provider that provides protection for medical expenses above a specified dollar amount.

Straw Man: An untrue version of the opposing view set up to gain a victory in debate or argumentation; this can be a demonized version of the opposition view or a weakened version of the opposing premise.

Sublimation: The satisfying of an unacceptable impulse indirectly by taking as its object a socially acceptable end

Target Market: The group of buyers (or potential buyers) that share common needs or characteristics, which the organization intends to serve.

Tax Subsidized: Economic circumstances where the federal government reduces the cost of a program or service by direct cash payments or through tax savings to the providers which permit the provider to reduce the cost of the program by the amount of any tax savings.

Telecommuting: A practice that allows employees to work from home and communicate with the office through phone, fax, e-mail or other forms of technology.

Turnover Rate: The percentage of employees who leave the organization over a given time period.

Quality: The degree to which a good or service meets established standards or satisfies the customer.

Quality Health Care: The appropriate care from qualified providers delivered in the most appropriate manner and setting for the patient's unique circumstances.

Withhold: The amount of a primary care physician's (PCPs) capitation or fee-for-service fee payment (usually a percentage of the capitation or a flat dollar amount) that is withheld by the plan until year-end and either used to pay for incentive payments and bonuses to PCPs or retained by the plan due to greater-than-expected use of services.